Cerebrovascular Diseases - Elucidating Key Principles

Edited by Patricia Bozzetto Ambrosi

Published in London, United Kingdom

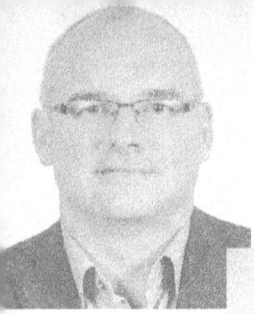
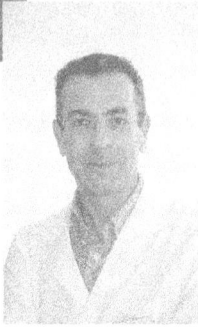
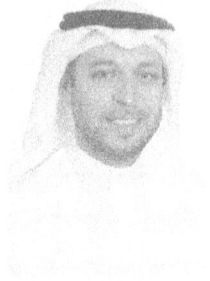
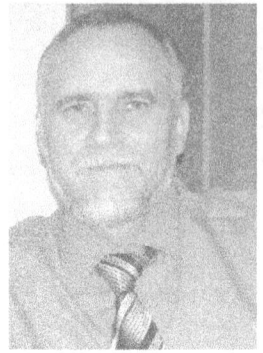
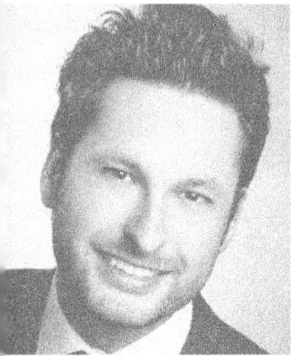
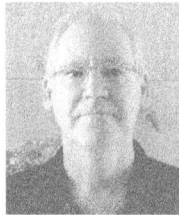
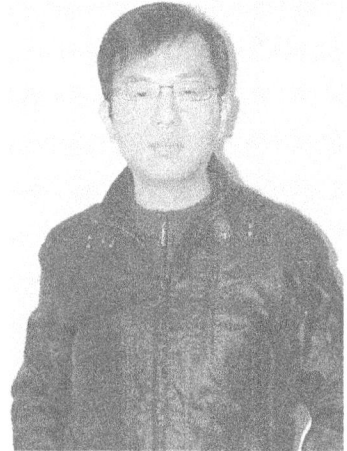

IntechOpen

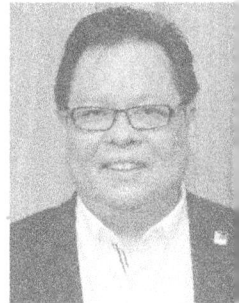
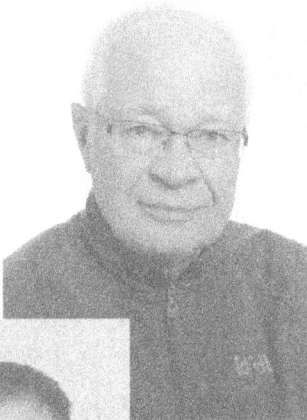
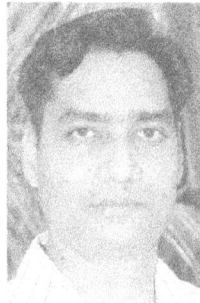
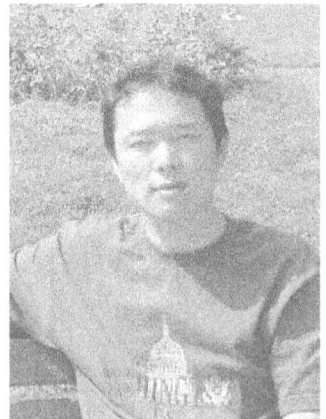
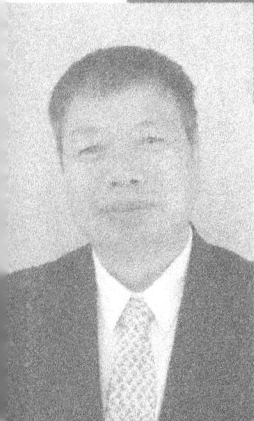
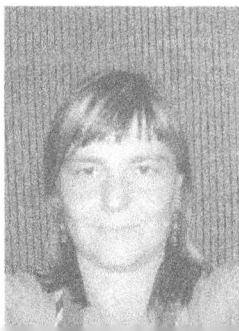

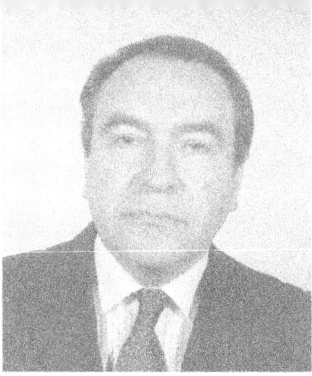

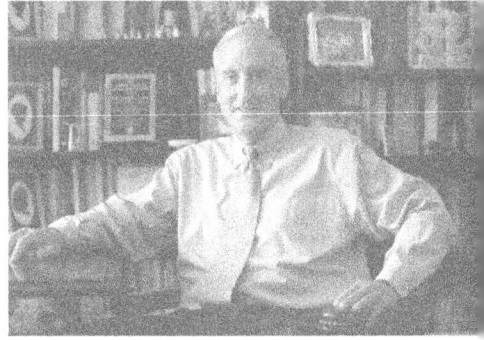

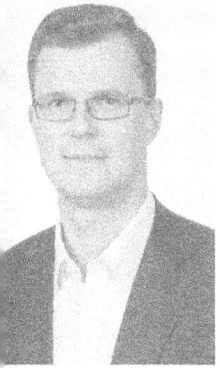

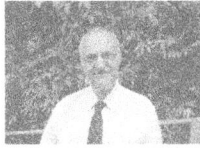

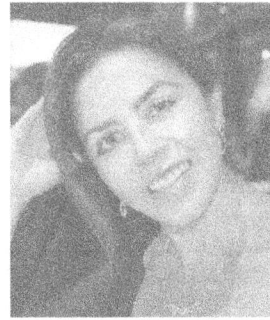

Supporting open minds since 2005

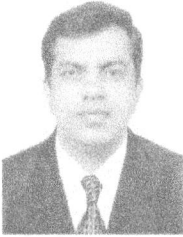

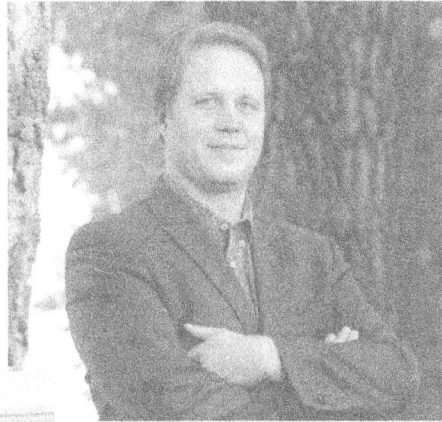

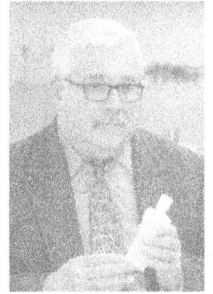

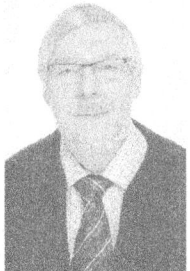

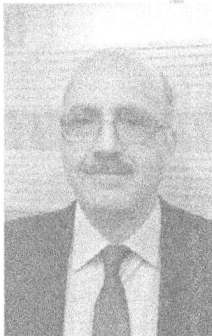

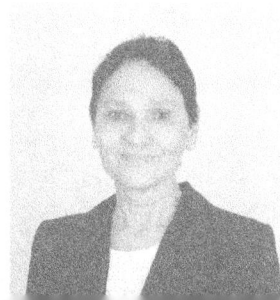

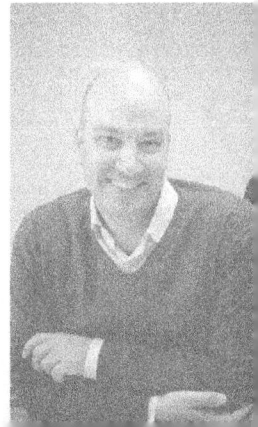

Cerebrovascular Diseases – Elucidating Key Principles
http://dx.doi.org/10.5772/intechopen.94805
Edited by Patricia Bozzetto Ambrosi

Contributors
Orleancio Gomes Ripardo de Azevedo, Rafael Costa Lima Maia, Henrique Coelho Silva, Paulo Roberto Leitao de Vasconcelos, María Cristina Zurrú, Marianela López Armaretti, Natalia Romina Balian, Irina Alexandrovna Savvina, Anna Olegovna Petrova, Yulia Mikhailovna Zabrodskaya, Konstantin Alexandrovich Samochernykh, Tecla Mlambo, Yvonne Pfavai, Faith R. Chimusoro, Farayi Kaseke, Gilberto Sousa Alves, Felipe Kenji Sudo, Santi Martini, Hermina Novida, Kuntoro, Mustafa Çetiner, Francesca Spagnolo, Vincenza Pinto, Augusto Maria Rini, Olga Razumnikova, Vladislav Kagan, Navdeep Singh Sidhu, Sumandeep Kaur

Notice
Statements and opinions expressed in the chapters are these of the individual contributors and not necessarily those of the editors or publisher. No responsibility is accepted for the accuracy of information contained in the published chapters. The publisher assumes no responsibility for any damage or injury to persons or property arising out of the use of any materials, instructions, methods or ideas contained in the book.

First published in London, United Kingdom, 2022 by IntechOpen
IntechOpen is the global imprint of INTECHOPEN LIMITED, registered in England and Wales, registration number: 11086078, 5 Princes Gate Court, London, SW7 2QJ, United Kingdom
Printed in Croatia

British Library Cataloguing-in-Publication Data
A catalogue record for this book is available from the British Library

Additional hard and PDF copies can be obtained from orders@intechopen.com

Cerebrovascular Diseases – Elucidating Key Principles
Edited by Patricia Bozzetto Ambrosi
p. cm.
Print ISBN 978-1-83962-700-2
Online ISBN 978-1-83962-701-9
eBook (PDF) ISBN 978-1-83962-702-6

We are IntechOpen,
the world's leading publisher of
Open Access books
Built by scientists, for scientists

6,000+
Open access books available

146,000+
International authors and editors

185M+
Downloads

Our authors are among the

156
Countries delivered to

Top 1%
most cited scientists

12.2%
Contributors from top 500 universities

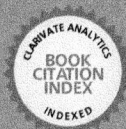

Interested in publishing with us?
Contact book.department@intechopen.com

Numbers displayed above are based on latest data collected.
For more information visit www.intechopen.com

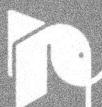

Meet the editor

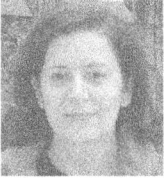

Prof. Dr. Patricia Bozzetto Ambrosi graduated in Medicine from the University of Caxias do Sul, Brazil, and the University of Rome Tor Vergata, Italy. She is a former researcher in morpho-physiology at the University of Córdoba/Reina Sofia Hospital, Spain. She graduated in Neurology/Neurosurgery at the Hospital of Restaura, SES, Brazil, and in Neuroradiology/Radiodiagnostics at Paris Marie Curie University, France. She holds a master's degree in Medicine from the University of Nova Lisboa, Portugal, and one in Behavioral Sciences and Neuropsychiatry from the University of Pernambuco, Brazil. She also has a Ph.D. in Biological Sciences from the University of Pernambuco/Paris Diderot University. She is a former fellow in Interventional Neuroradiology at the Ophthalmological Foundation Adolphe de Rothschild, Beaujon Hospital, and Hospices Civils de Strasbourg, France. She was a praticien associe in Interventional Neuroradiology at Neurologique Hospital Pierre Wertheimer, University of Lyon Claude Bernard, France, and a visiting professor at the University of Paris Diderot-Neuri Beaujon. She is an independent consultant/supervisor in neuroradiology, neuroendovascular, and imaging and a clinical professor of medicine. She has been an academic collaborator researcher in the Cardiovascular Department, University of Leicester, England. Dr. Ambrosi has experience in innovative research for the development of new technologies and neurosciences and is an academic editor and reviewer of several scientific publications about neurological diseases.

Contents

Preface

Among all neurological diseases, cerebrovascular diseases (CVDs) stand out for their considerable frequency. They are a leading cause of death for both men and women. A stroke is the sudden onset of a focal neurologic deficit. Strokes are categorized as ischemic or hemorrhagic, with the former being due to occlusion of a blood vessel and the latter being due to bursting of a blood vessel. The resulting neurological syndrome corresponds to a portion of the brain that is supplied by one or more cerebral vessels, resulting in stroke syndromes.

This book discusses the fundamental principles of cerebrovascular diseases. Chapter 1 presents aspects of inflammatory and oxidative stress associated with CVDs, focusing on biomarkers. It also examines the role of omega oils and the intracellular molecular network associated with tissue load in these conditions. Chapter 2 deals with CVD and hypertension, particularly systemic hypertension, which is a major public health problem affecting nearly one-third of the global adult population. It is the main modifiable risk factor for vascular diseases leading to considerable degrees of morbidity and mortality. A large body of clinical evidence has shown that adequate control of high blood pressure can be a very effective tool in reducing the incidence and prevalence of CVDs. Chapter 3 discusses atrial fibrillation, which is one of the main causes of morbidity and mortality in adults, especially due to its strong association with stroke. The chapter presents the typical clinical and radiological features of cardioembolic strokes, addressing acute reperfusion therapies. Chapter 4 discusses cryptogenic stroke (CS), which is a challenging pathology responsible for approximately 30%–40% of all ischemic strokes. Despite being defined as the presence of cerebral infarctions, a cause that was not identified despite an adequate diagnostic evaluation, there is a certain subgroup of CS with embolic features in neuroimaging studies and without evidence of alternative atrial fibrillation or any alternative cause. Therefore, the chapter reviews information on the rationale and data behind the pathophysiology, proposed biomarkers, and therapeutic implications of CS. Despite being defined as the presence of cerebral infarctions, a cause that was not identified despite an adequate diagnostic evaluation, there is a certain subgroup of CS with embolic features in neuroimaging studies and without evidence of alternative atrial fibrillation or any alternative cause, therefore we reviewed information on the rationale and data behind its pathophysiology, proposed biomarkers of atrial heart disease, and therapeutic implications in cerebrovascular disease. Chapter 5 discusses cerebrovascular diseases as an important cause of dementia. Their presence, isolated or associated with degenerative conditions, increases the risk of conversion to progressive cognitive decline, with neuropsychiatric manifestations varying according to the affected brain territory and the disrupted neuronal circuits. The chapter also explores diagnostic and therapeutic approaches, including preventive and health promotion strategies for timely management of vascular risk factors and symptomatic approaches. Chapter 6 discusses cerebral vasospasm, which is a major cause of mortality and disability in patients with acute cerebral circulatory disorders. Chapter 7 reviews and addresses reperfusion therapies with a focus on intravenous thrombolytic therapy, one of the reperfusion therapies applied in the acute phase of stroke. Chapter 8 deals with infarction stroke and blood glucose associated with food consumption in Indonesia. Chapter 9 shows that there is an age-associated specificity in the temporal dynamics of changes in visual-spatial short-term memory. It also highlights the considerable success of systematic long-term visual-spatial memory training in old age. Finally, Chapter 10 concludes by presenting an overview of stroke and rehabilitation with a specific emphasis on occupational therapy. It discusses the activities and areas of participation considered important by stroke patients, their needs, and the perceived satisfaction of these needs to provide targeted interventions. It also presents the results of studies conducted in Zimbabwe.

Dr. Patricia Bozzetto Ambrosi
Professor,
Independent Neuroradiologist Consultant,
Clinical Professor and Academic Researcher,
Fellow of European Academy of Neurology,
London, United Kingdom

Section 1

Pathophysiology

Chapter 1

The Pathophysiological Aspects of Cerebral Diseases

Henrique Coelho Silva, Rafael Costa Lima Maia,
Paulo Roberto Leitao de Vasconcelos
and Orleancio Gomes Ripardo de Azevedo

Abstract

Introduction. Cerebrovascular disorders are the main causes of heavy burden health worldwide, also, it is critical to understand the pathophysiological mechanism and then trying to prevent the neurological sequels. **Objective**. To discuss the inflammatory and oxidative stress aspects associated to the cerebrovascular diseases, focusing on biomarkers, also the role of omega oils, and the intracellular molecular network associated to the tissue burden on those conditions. **Results**. One of the most promising biomarkers it is Neuron-Specific Enolase (NSE). Serum NSE levels were elevated in stroke-patients compared to the non-stroke controls. Also, studies have demonstrated that in specific ratio omega oils 3, 6 and 9 can ameliorate the inflammatory and oxidative stress in nervous tissue and could be useful to the inflammatory and oxidative stress negative effects of cerebrovascular diseases. In addition, the study of the molecular mechanisms is essential to understand which molecules could be addressed in cascade of events preventing the permanent damage on the nervous tissue. **Final considerations**. The studies on cerebrovascular disorders must precisely identify the mechanisms and key molecules involved and improve the time of diagnostics and prognostics reducing the negative impacts of those conditions.

Keywords: Neuroinflammation, oxidative stress, omega oils, biomarkers, molecular Cascade, pathophysiology

1. Introduction

Cerebrovascular disease is an important cause of severe health impairment and/or death, being the stroke, the main event-related as a cause of this group of diseases. The American Association of Neurological Surgeons (AANS) define cerebrovascular disease as disorder, in which, an area of the brain is temporarily or permanently affected by ischemia or bleeding and one or more of the cerebral blood vessels are involved in the pathological process, which includes stroke, carotid stenosis, vertebral and intracranial stenosis, aneurysms, and vascular malformations [1].

Other conditions such as brain tumors, neurotrauma, intracerebral hematoma, and aneurysmal subarachnoid hemorrhage, could be potentially important depending on the incidence or prevalence in populations across the world [2]. Cerebrovascular diseases are frequently associated with the high financial cost to the public and private health system across developed and under-resourced countries.

2. Expenditures for cerebrovascular disease patients

Brazil has shown a high level of economic burden to manage and treat cerebrovascular diseases. In a Brazilian report, the authors have demonstrated the annual costs and use of health care compared, age and sex paired healthy individuals to patients with cerebrovascular disease [3].

Reis Neto and Busch evaluated the annual costs and the use of private health care systems comparing 71,094 individuals among healthy controls and patients with cerebrovascular conditions. The 12 months follow-up report, found that the annual individual expenditure was 65.6% higher compared to the control group without any cerebrovascular condition [3].

Several reports have demonstrated that the main cause of cerebrovascular disease is stroke, which leads to a huge impact on brain tissue due to restriction on blood flow compromising the nervous tissue and leading to negative effects.

3. Stroke

According to the World Health Organization (WHO), stroke is a condition that the blood flow is interrupted leading to a focal or global disturbance on brain functions showing symptoms during at least 24 hours or longer or even leading to the death of the patient [4].

3.1 Types of strokes

Since the stroke is related to the blood flow to the nervous tissue, the stroke could be divided into (1) ischemic stroke and (2) hemorrhagic stroke.

The ischemic stroke resulted in obstruction of a large vessel in the brain or cervical region leading to reduced levels of oxygen and glucose diffusion to the after-occlusion regions, particularly classified in two regions—*penumbra* and *ischemic core* (**Figure 1**) with some important characteristics. On the other hand, hemorrhagic stroke is produced due to a rupture of a vessel mainly due to hypertensive disease, coagulation disorders vascular malformation and could be potentialized by diet and other modifiable factors [4].

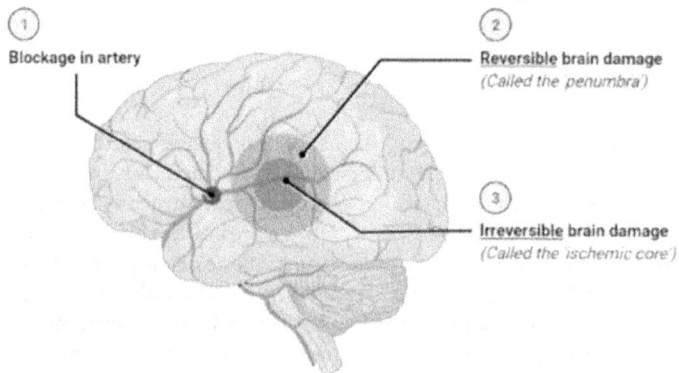

Figure 1.
A schematic illustration for brain damage provoked by an ischemic stroke (created with BioRender.com®).

Worldwide in 2016, there were 5.5 million deaths related to the consequences of stroke, in addition, 80.1 million prevalent cases, being 41.1 and 39.0 in female and male respectively, also 13.7 million new cases of stroke cases worldwide [5].

The last published 2021 guideline for the prevention of stroke summarizes the types and subtypes of stroke (**Figure 2**) according to the anatomy location and involvement [6–8]. Those phenotypes are key features to provide accurate information to the physician to take a correct decision and may deliver a proper assistance to the patients.

In the acute phase of cerebral arterial occlusion, the critical treatment consists of recovering cerebral reperfusion as soon as possible. Currently, two therapies are validated for this purpose—intravenous thrombolytic (rtPA) and/or mechanical thrombectomy [9].

Each of these modalities has advantages and disadvantages. However, less than 20% of all stroke patients are candidates for mechanical thrombectomy, making primary and secondary prevention still the major factors to reduce the number of cases in the world. The prevention of stroke is based on a healthy diet, regular exercise, and avoiding smoking and alcohol consumption.

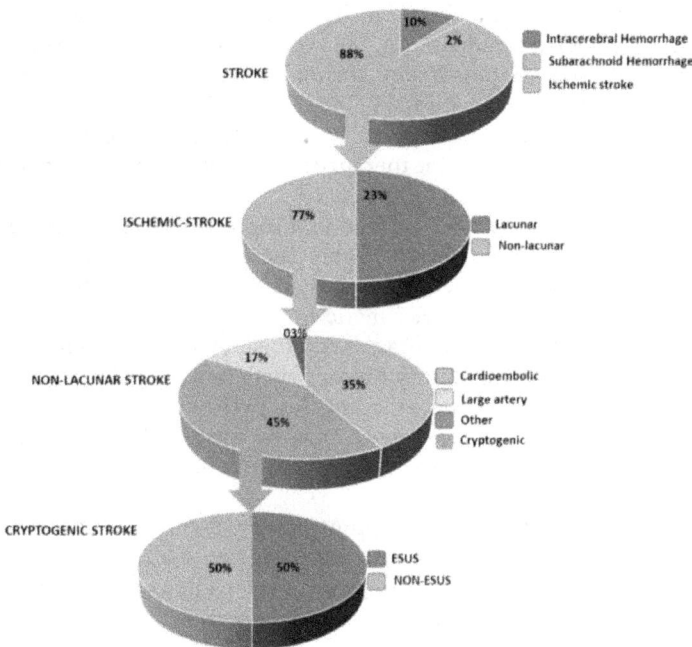

Figure 2.
The classification of stroke subtypes according to the definition and anatomical localization (created with BioRender.com®).

3.2 Pathophysiology of stroke

In ischemic stroke, an interruption in cellular oxidative metabolism decreases the oxidative metabolism, levels of calcium and sodium, these key factors lead to a reduction in oxygen-based neuronal mitochondrial function, energetic debit, production, and releasing of inflammatory mediators (prostaglandin and leukotrienes), in addition, vasoconstriction, platelet aggregation, and vessel occlusion.

On the other hand, a hemorrhagic cerebrovascular event, an acute vessel rupture of encephalic structures; a secondary ischemic lesion around the hematoma may also occur [10–12].

The anti-inflammatory and antioxidative roles of omega oils 3, 6, and 9 have been largely investigated in cerebrovascular diseases [13–15].

The economical, epidemiological, and pathophysiology impacts of cerebrovascular diseases are huge and must be addressed to improve the comprehension of all the factors that are related to the genesis and the disease progression of these conditions. Thus, the animal models could be potentially positive helping to clarify all the key factors related to cerebrovascular diseases.

3.3 Inflammatory and oxidative state in stroke

Several studies have been conducted in the past to assess the benefit of cerebral arterial reperfusion, but only in 1995, the benefit was proven using intravenous thrombolysis with alteplase (tPA) to break the cerebral thrombus [16].

A recent report has suggested superiority in treatment with a new clot buster "tenecteplase" (TNK), a variant of tPA, but possesses greater fibrin specificity and a longer half-life, making it potentially safer and a more effective drug for stroke [17]. In addition to intravenous thrombolytic therapy, the treatment of patients with stroke is having profound modifications due to the endovascular treatment of cerebral reperfusion, increasing the therapeutic window for up to 24 hours from the onset of initial symptoms [18].

Early treatment is the most critical factor for successful reperfusion therapy of acute ischemic stroke. The researchers only discovered the correct way to treat stroke patients in the acute phase after understanding exactly how the alteration in cerebral blood flow modifies the cell function.

Acute occlusion of an arterial branch responsible for the irrigation of a brain area triggers an inflammatory cascade that clinically manifests as an acute neurological deficit. However, according to the degree of dependence of that cell on the vessel, different metabolic responses will occur. The brain requires a continuous supply of oxygen and glucose to maintain physiologic function.

The regular brain perfusion rate is approximately 50–60 mL/100 g tissue/min, if cerebral blood flow is interrupted, then neuronal metabolism can be affected after 30 seconds of interruption and will completely stop within 2 minutes of deprivation. Through the increase in the cellular capacity to extract oxygen under low supply conditions, no symptoms are observed until the brain blood flow reaches around 20–30 mL/100 g/min [19], and then the energy generation is shifted to the anaerobic glycolysis pathway.

This is the basis of the glutamate excitotoxicity theory and may explain why pyramidal neurons in the hippocampus and Purkinje cells in the cerebellum that rely on glutamate neurotransmission are particularly vulnerable to ischemia [20]. The center of the irrigated tissue area, when receiving less than 10 ml/100 g of brain tissue, after 4–5 minutes, cannot maintain the sodium and potassium transporter working, generating a cytotoxic edema that will evolve to cell apoptosis, a process mediated by calcium and the glutamate (**Figure 3**) [21].

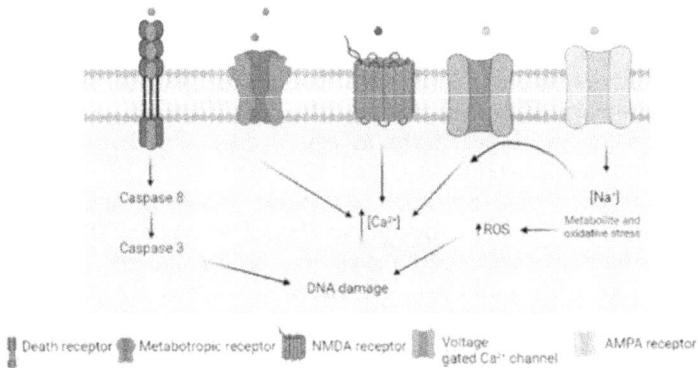

Figure 3.
Molecular pathways outlining the role of glutamate in excitotoxicity following stroke (created with BioRender.com®).

3.4 Stroke blood biomarkers

One of the major difficulties for the acute treatment of patients with cerebral ischemia is early diagnosis through a serum biomarker since stroke often occurs with atypical and nonspecific symptoms, known as *"stroke chameleons"* [22].

The biomarker must be reliable, rapidly measured, and readily available, to be considered a good biomarker for stroke. In addition, the biomarker must help in determining the mechanism of injury, differentiating in cardioembolic, atherothrombotic, or prothrombotic state [23].

However, the stroke biomarkers do not have sufficient data to support an ideal concept of sensitivity and specificity [24] to standard any biomarker by itself to characterize the progression of the disease. In addition, Lassen, and cols., first reported that acute occlusion of an arterial branch responsible for the irrigation of a brain area triggers an inflammatory cascade that clinically manifests as an acute neurological deficit. However, different metabolic responses will occur leading to difficulty to identify a biomarker that shows specificity and sensibility for a lab detection [19].

One of the most promising markers evaluated is neuron-specific enolase (NSE), an enzyme released after neuronal damage. Serum NSE levels were elevated in stroke patients compared to the nonstroke controls and are associated with infarct volume and high neurological deficit [25]. Nonetheless, the NSE major issue to be standardized as a biomarker is delayed-release into the blood flow after brain injury compromising, the key role of early diagnosis [26].

Furthermore, the brain natriuretic peptide (BNP) is the main cardiac biomarker studied for its relationship with stroke, including the presence of paroxysmal atrial fibrillation, although optimal cutoff values for individual profiles are undefined [27].

In addition, studies from a European consortium of the population-based cohort (approximately 58.000 stroke-free participants), evaluating brain natriuretic peptide (BNP) levels, demonstrated that increased levels of NT-proBNP were associated with the higher risk of ischemic and hemorrhagic stroke [28].

Another study assessing 381 patients diagnosed with the transient ischemic attack (TIA), has shown an NT-proBNP level > 800 pg./mL, which was independently associated with a higher risk of stroke over 37 months follow-up [29].

4. Animals models in cerebrovascular diseases

The pathophysiology of cerebrovascular diseases such as ischemia has been studied in several animal models. These models have shown many metabolic alterations leading to cellular lesions in specific brain regions, depending on the duration of the blood flow restriction [10–12].

The use of small animals (e.g., mice, rats, gerbils, or rabbits) have an important advantage; lower maintenance costs compared to larger animals. The rat is the most used in stoke studies, due to the physiology and anatomy similarity to the humans [30], however, the mouse could be potentially useful, since is the uses of transgenic technology that can assess the molecular pathophysiology of stroke [31, 32].

The middle cerebral artery permanent or transient occlusion (MCAo) is less invasive and does not require craniectomy and has been widely used in published reports. In the transient method, the duration of suture varies between 60 and 120 minutes inducing high levels of infarction (**Figure 4**) [33].

The photothrombosis model is based on intravascular oxidation through irradiation with a light beam in a specific wavelength, generating oxygen radicals that lead to inflammation-like damage [34]. The Endothelin-1, a potent vasoconstrictor, it is administered in the Middle of Cerebral Artery (MCA) leading to the animal develops stroke.

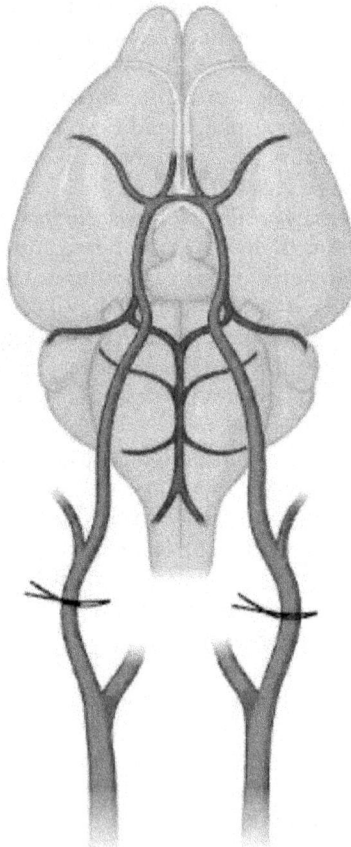

Bilateral occlusion of
common carotid arteries

Figure 4.
The representation of bilateral occlusion of common carotid arteries. (created with BioRender.com®).

Another model is the embolic stroke that uses clots with spheres of dextran or other supraparamagnetic iron oxides, TiO_2, and ceramic that could develop occlusion and lead to stroke [35].

In the last years of animal models to understand the mechanisms involved in stroke, it is widely used to evaluate key targets and therapeutics molecules investigating the protectives and treatments tools. The administration of omega 3, 6, and 9 could be a useful tool to protect the nervous tissue against the inflammatory and oxidative damages produced by stroke [33–35].

4.1 Use of omega, 3, 6 and 9 in brain ischemia animal models

The brain ischemia leads to several metabolic alterations in carbohydrates metabolism in an experimental model of brain ischemia-induced only by the bilateral occlusion of common carotid arteries in rats [36].

However, some evidence suggests that ketone bodies are utilized to generate energy in some extreme situations such as ischemia [37]. In addition, in a report from Faria and cols in 2007, the authors have demonstrated, that using 48 male Wistar rats submitted to the occlusion of common carotid arteries, increased cerebral uptake of acetoacetate (ACT) and beta-hydroxybutyrate (BHB) following brain ischemia [38].

Pinheiro and cols in 2011, have shown that the preconditioning of 42 male rats with different omega oil mix preparations promoted protection against the deleterious effects of ischemia/reperfusion injury demonstrated by the reduction of red neurons in the group that received mix 2 (omega 6: omega 3 ratio— 1.4:1; omega 9: omega 6 ratio—3.4:1) source of omega 3 ALA (35%) + EPA (39%) + DHA (26%) [39].

In 2011 Campelo et al., using occlusion of the common bilateral carotid arteries ischemia model demonstrated that the pretreatment using nitrosyl-ruthenium (Rut-bpy) decreased the mean arterial pressure variations throughout the transition of brain ischemia to reperfusion, in addition, decreased the ischemic area, also Rut-bpy pretreatment reduced NF-kB hippocampal immunostaining and protein expression with improved histopathology scoring as compared to the untreated ischemic-group control [40].

Pires and colleagues in 2011, using the L-Ala-Gln preconditioned gerbils (*Meriones unguiculatus*) under the transient bilateral occlusion of the common carotid arteries, demonstrated a significant increased GSH levels [41]. Furthermore, Oliveira and cols. Demonstrated an important reduction on TNF-α, NF-κB, IL-6, and HO-1, inflammatory mediators in pretreated gerbils with L-Ala-Gln [42].

5. The pathophysiology of subarachnoid hemorrhage

In addition to stoke, the role of the oxidative state in the context of subarachnoid hemorrhage is another fascinating topic that deserves to be studied.

The incidence of delayed cerebral ischemia (DCI) is around 30%, with DCI remaining the major cause of morbidity and mortality among patients who survive the initial treatment of the ruptured aneurysm [43]. The DCI is frequently associated with the early arteriolar vasospasm with microthrombosis, perfusion difficulty and neurovascular uncoupling, spreading neurons depolarizations, and inflammatory responses that begin at the time of the aneurysmal subarachnoid hemorrhage (aSAH) and evolve over time, culminating in cortical infarction [44].

The aSAH (approximately the origin of 5% of all strokes) is a complex cerebrovascular disease with severe systemic complications. The worldwide incidence of aSAH is approximately 700,000 cases annually with a mortality rate of about 40% [45].

The initial global hypoperfusion after aSAH leads to inflammatory processes, which occur in blood vessels as well as in cerebrospinal fluid (CSF) and then macrophages and neutrophils enter the subarachnoid space releasing proinflammatory factors [46].

The initial aneurysmal rupture deposits blood within the subarachnoid space, the methemoglobin, heme, and hemin resulting from red blood cell breakdown and hemoglobin metabolism, which can lead to activation of TLR4, which stimulates a pro-inflammatory cascade damaging neurons and white matter. Hemin has been associated with the release of redox-active iron, which depletes antioxidant stores, such as, nicotinamide adenine dinucleotide phosphate (NADPH) and glutathione while producing superoxide and hydroxyl radicals as well as increasing lipid peroxidation [47].

Some clinical studies have found that modulating inflammation following aSAH is beneficial, on the other hand, several studies have shown, no beneficial effect at all. It is likely that activation of inflammation at different time points post rupture, is associated with different protective or detrimental responses depending on the microenvironment and type of cells recruited to the inflammatory site [48].

One of the most commonly proinflammatory biomarkers used as a clinical indicator of its C-reactive protein (CRP), that plays an important role in disease diagnosis and treatment and management evaluation. Recent research has shown that CRP (C-reactive protein) is an independent predictor of outcome after aSAH [49].

In a study conducted from January 2012 to June 2017, developed in South Korea, the researchers evaluating 156 patients diagnosed with aSAH found, evidence that serial measurements of CRP may be used to predict neurological outcomes of SAH patients, in addition, maximal CRP levels within 4 days post-SAH are significantly correlated with poor neurological outcomes [50].

Injection of proinflammatory components induces cerebral vasospasm, even in the absence of blood breakdown products (**Figure 5**) [48].

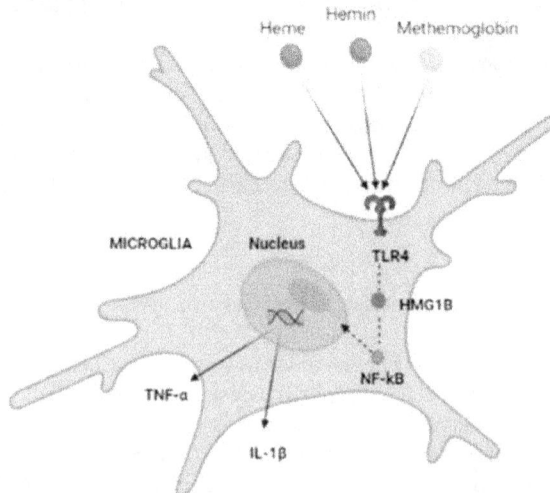

Figure 5.
The damage in red blood cells, led to the release of molecules such as heme, hemin, and methemoglobin, through the TLR4, activating the group box 1 genes and then leading to the production and releasing of proinflammatory molecules TNF-α and NF-κB [51] (created with BioRender.com®).

Clinically, the inflammatory response appears in close temporal relationship with the spasm and direct proportion to the magnitude of the inflammatory response [52]. These findings have been supported by evidence suggesting that the accumulation of inflammatory cells closely parallels neuronal cell death. Cell death near the vasculature has been substantially reduced by the depletion of inflammatory cells in preclinical studies [53].

One of the main lines of research related to aSAH is the identification of a specific biomarker related to the risk of a patient presenting late cerebral ischemia, allowing anticipation of specific therapy for the condition.

The difficulty in using biomarkers in clinical practice stems from the variability of inflammatory markers according to the phase of hemorrhage, which can protect the brain tissue in a certain phase and attack the brain tissue in another phase. In addition, the high financial, temporal, and human cost of measuring these markers makes them unfeasible, currently, for routine clinical use [54].

6. Inflammatory and oxidative state in brain tumors

Other types of brain lesions, in addition to primarily vascular ones, have inflammatory and oxidative aspects in pathogenesis. We will initially discuss brain tumors, and the next topic, brain trauma.

The importance of the inflammatory state in oncological diseases in the central nervous system (CNS) is already well established and valued. Even with damage to other systems, there are changes in the neuroinflammatory microenvironment induced by the underlying oncological disease that is reflected in the functioning of the CNS [55–57].

Primary tumors of the nervous system are strongly related to the production of reactive oxygen species (ROS), promoting abnormalities in DNA replication, activating of proinflammatory gene panel, and subsequent inflammation in the tumor microenvironment [58], which is reflected, for example, in the presence of tumor-associated macrophages (TAM's), which arise specifically from microglia in the context of gliomas [59, 60].

Presenting all proinflammatory-related genes, cytokines, and mediators involved in this state is beyond the scope of this chapter. However, this proinflammatory state has been present since the first stages of tumorigenesis [61] and can be fed back by the glioma cells themselves, as demonstrated by Lisi 2014 *et al.*, who pointed out that brain tumor gene expression varies throughout the natural history of the disease, mainly alternating the expression of M1 and M2a/B, promoting the release of different growth factors according to the stages of advancement [62].

This "phenotypic shift" is also implicated in disrupting the natural cycle of microglial mitosis [63]. We should also discuss the key role of external elements, such as Benzo[a]pyrene, promoting oxidative stress, leading the DNA damage arising from DNA mutations. On the other hand, Patri 2019 *et al* suggest that noradrenaline may have a protective effect against this effect [64].

Feng 2020 demonstrated through enrichment levels of 28 immune cells in the tumor immune microenvironment in five datasets, demonstrating prognostic (and consequent therapeutic) implications through phenomena that diverge from those observed in other types of cancer. The phenotype involved, for example, allows the tumor to evade the immune response mechanism [65]. Among the ways to exercise this immune-resistant condition can be cited suppression of EZH2 [66] and T cell dysfunction promoting the sustained growth of the tumor [67, 68].

The understanding of neuroinflammatory implications extends beyond the formulation of specific therapies to combat the growth and perpetuation of the neoplasm—oxidative stress has a strong influence on the outcome also in the postoperative state of tumor resection, and the correct conduct with this in mind can also influence the outcome [69].

7. Inflammatory and oxidative state in traumatic brain injury (TBI)

TBI is one of the main causes of brain damage, especially in the young population. The cumulation of inflammatory factors is associated with the increased tissue damage of the nervous system in both the brain and spinal cord [70], causing lesions through ischemic-like patterns mechanisms [71].

In the initial moments, proinflammatory cytokines IL-1α, IL-1β, IL-6, and TNF-α, are released in sustained-response patter reaching and activating the microglia, being predominant during the first 48 hours [70, 72, 73].

Even in cases of mild traumatic brain injury, which commonly do not present with more exuberant clinical conditions, there is evidence of neuroinflammation, and apoptosis related to oxidative stress [74].

Interestingly, there is evidence for similar patterns in psychiatric conditions where trauma itself is not (or at least is not sustained) the main factor involved, as in post-traumatic stress disorder [75, 76]. Hyperfibrinogenemia is another common factor in the proinflammatory state of TBI and other neurological conditions such as Alzheimer's disease [77].

Among the substances studied in this context is the release of nitric oxide (NO), produced by endothelial nitric oxide synthase [78]. Abdul-Muneer 2014 described the interactions involved between several inflammatory cytokines and growth factors involved in oxidative stress and neurovascular inflammation in the pathogenesis of TBI, highlighting blood–brain barrier dysfunction (BBB) in the onset and perpetuation of changes in the cellular microenvironment in this pathological condition [79].

Recognition of the role of the inflammatory microenvironment, both in the acute and later phases of TBI, offers a therapeutic opportunity by changing the phenotype from proinflammatory to anti-inflammatory, which represents the fertile area for research [74, 80]. Chemokines are emerging as powerful controlling inflammation-induced brain edema factors, especially regarding BBB dysfunction [81]. In another example, there is evidence that hypothermia can be used to curb the inflammatory cascade [70].

8. Closing remarks

Thus, the research of neurovascular diseases, as well as the understanding of other brain injuries initially nonvascular (such as neoplasms and traumas) should identify the critical molecules of the cascade of the disease mechanism that could be potentially used, such as, a biomarker and used to develops prognostics to understand how the disease progression is. On the other hand, as fast as, the inflammatory and oxidative mechanisms are revealed; more and more molecules can be used as therapeutical tools to address the negative clinical signs associated with disease.

Acknowledgements

The authors would like to be thankful to the surgery department of the Federal University of Ceara, for the entire support for the development of their studies and move forward on elucidating those very critical conditions that affect the population.

The Pathophysiological Aspects of Cerebral Diseases
DOI: http://dx.doi.org/10.5772/intechopen.101218

Conflict of interest

The authors declare no conflict of interest.

Author details

Henrique Coelho Silva[1], Rafael Costa Lima Maia[2],
Paulo Roberto Leitao de Vasconcelos[2]
and Orleancio Gomes Ripardo de Azevedo[2]*

1 General Hospital of Fortaleza, Fortaleza, Brazil

2 Surgery Department, Federal University of Ceara, Fortaleza, Brazil

*Address all correspondence to: orleancio@gmail.com

IntechOpen

References

[1] Neurosurgical Conditions and Treatments. American Association of Neurological Surgeons; 2021. Available from: https://www.aans.org/en/Patients/Neurosurgical-Conditions-and-Treatments/Cerebrovascular-Disease [Accessed: 09/05/2021]

[2] Pan P et al. A review of hematoma components clearance mechanism after subarachnoid hemorrhage. Frontiers in Neuroscience. 2020;**14**:1-10. DOI: 10.3389/fnins.2020.00685

[3] Reis Neto JP, Busch J. PCV148 Estimate of the impact and costs of cerebrovascular disease from a health plan in brazil: Real world scenario study. Value in Health. 2019;**22**:S569. DOI: 10.1016/j.jval.2019.09.872

[4] Aho K, Harmsen P, Hatano S, Marquardsen J, Smirnov VE, Strasser T. Cerebrovascular disease in the community: Results of a WHO collaborative study. Bulletin of the World Health Organization. 1980;**58**:113-130

[5] Johnson CO et al. Global, regional, and national burden of stroke, 1990-2016: A systematic analysis for the Global Burden of Disease Study 2016. The Lancet Neurology. 2019;**18**(5): 439-458. DOI: 10.1016/S1474-4422 (19)30034-1

[6] Kolominsky-Rabas PL, Weber M, Gefeller O, Neundoerfer B, Heuschmann PU. Epidemiology of ischemic stroke subtypes according to TOAST Criteria. Stroke. 2001; **32**(12):2735-2740. DOI: 10.1161/hs1201.100209

[7] Gardener H, Sacco RL, Rundek T, Battistella V, Cheung YK, Elkind MSV. Race and ethnic disparities in stroke incidence in the Northern Manhattan Study. Stroke. 2020;**51**(4):1064-1069. DOI: 10.1161/STROKEAHA.119.028806

[8] Adams HP et al. Classification of subtype of acute ischemic stroke. Definitions for use in a multicenter clinical trial. TOAST. Trial of Org 10172 in Acute Stroke Treatment. Stroke. 1993;**24**(1):35-41. DOI: 10.1161/01. STR.24.1.35

[9] Kleindorfer DO et al. 2021 Guideline for the prevention of stroke in patients with stroke and transient ischemic attack: A guideline from the american heart association/american stroke association. Stroke. 2021;**52**(7): e364–e467. DOI: 10.1161/STR. 0000000000000375

[10] Farooqui AA, Hann SE, Horrocks LA. Basic neurochemistry: Molecular, cellular and medical aspects. In: Siegel GJ, Agranoff BW, Albers RW, Fisher SK, Uhler MD, editors. Basic Neurochemistry, Molecular, Cellular and Medical Aspects. 6th ed. New York: Lippincott-Raven; 1999

[11] Homi HM, da Silva Júnior BA, Velasco IT. Fisiopatologia da Isquemia Cerebral. Revista Brasileira de Anestesiologia. 2000;**50**(5):405-414

[12] Molinari GF. Why model strokes? Stroke. 1988;**19**(10):1195-1197. DOI: 10.1161/01.STR.19.10.1195

[13] Shirley R, Ord E, Work L. Oxidative stress and the use of antioxidants in stroke. Antioxidants. 2014;**3**(3):472-501. DOI: 10.3390/antiox3030472

[14] Ueda M, Inaba T, Nito C, Kamiya N, Katayama Y. Therapeutic impact of eicosapentaenoic acid on ischemic brain damage following transient focal cerebral ischemia in rats. Brain Research. 2013;**1519**:95-104. DOI: 10.1016/j.brainres.2013.04.046

[15] Mozaffarian D, Micha R, Wallace S. Effects on coronary heart disease of Increasing polyunsaturated fat in place

of saturated fat: A systematic review and meta-analysis of randomized controlled trials. PLoS Medicine. 2010;**7**(3):1-10. DOI: 10.1371/journal.pmed.1000252

[16] National Institute of Neurological Disorders and Stroke rt-PA Stroke Study Group. Tissue plasminogen activator for acute ischemic stroke. New England Journal of Medicine. 1995;**333**(24):1581-1587. DOI: 10.1056/NEJM199512143332401

[17] Campbell BCV et al. Tenecteplase versus alteplase before thrombectomy for ischemic stroke. New England Journal of Medicine. 2018;**378**(17):1573-1582. DOI: 10.1056/NEJMoa1716405

[18] Nogueira RG et al. Thrombectomy 6 to 24 hours after stroke with a mismatch between deficit and infarct. New England Journal of Medicine. 2018;**378**(1). DOI: 10.1056/NEJMoa1706442

[19] Lassen NA. Cerebral blood flow and oxygen consumption in man. Physiological Reviews. 1959;**39**(2):11-21. DOI: 10.1152/physrev.1959.39.2.183

[20] Olney JW. Brain lesions, obesity, and other disturbances in mice treated with monosodium glutamate. Science. 1969;**164**(3880):719-21. DOI: 10.1126/science.164.3880.719

[21] Ansari J, Gavins FNE. The impact of thrombo-inflammation on the cerebral microcirculation. Microcirculation. 2021;**28**(3):1-11. DOI: 10.1111/micc.12689

[22] Dupre CM, Libman R, Dupre SI, Katz JM, Rybinnik I, Kwiatkowski T. Stroke Chameleons. Journal of Stroke and Cerebrovascular Diseases. 2014;**23**(2):374-8. DOI: 10.1016/j.jstrokecerebrovasdis.2013.07.015

[23] Dagonnier M, Donnan GA, Davis SM, Dewey HM, Howells DW.

Acute stroke biomarkers: Are we there yet? Frontiers in Neurology. 2021;**12**:1-16. DOI: 10.3389/fneur.2021.619721

[24] Whiteley W, Tseng M-C, Sandercock P. Blood biomarkers in the diagnosis of ischemic stroke. Stroke. 2008;**39**(10):2902-9. DOI: 10.1161/STROKEAHA.107.511261

[25] Anand N, Stead LG. Neuron-specific enolase as a marker for acute ischemic stroke: A systematic review. Cerebrovascular Diseases. 2005;**20**(4):213-219. DOI: 10.1159/000087701

[26] González-García S et al. Serum neuron-specific enolase and S100 calcium binding protein B biomarker levels do not improve diagnosis of acute stroke. The Journal of the Royal College of Physicians of Edinburgh. 2012;**42**(3):199-204. DOI: 10.4997/JRCPE.2012.302

[27] Cushman M et al. N-terminal pro–B-type natriuretic peptide and stroke risk. Stroke. 2014;**45**(6):1646-1650. DOI: 10.1161/STROKEAHA.114.004712

[28] di Castelnuovo A et al. NT-proBNP (N-terminal pro-B-type natriuretic peptide) and the risk of stroke. Stroke. 2019;**50**(3):610-617. DOI: 10.1161/STROKEAHA.118.023218

[29] Rodríguez-Castro E et al. NT-pro-BNP: A novel predictor of stroke risk after transient ischemic attack. International Journal of Cardiology. 2020;**298**:93-97. DOI: 10.1016/j.ijcard.2019.06.056

[30] Yamori Y, Horie R, Handa H, Sato M, Fukase M. Pathogenetic similarity of strokes in stroke-prone spontaneously hypertensive rats and humans. Stroke. 1976;**7**(1):46-53. DOI: 10.1161/01.STR.7.1.46

[31] Kraft P et al. FTY720 Ameliorates acute ischemic stroke in mice by

reducing thrombo-inflammation but not by direct neuroprotection. Stroke. 2013;**44**(11):3202-3210. DOI: 10.1161/ STROKEAHA.113.002880

[32] Göb E et al. Blocking of plasma kallikrein ameliorates stroke by reducing thromboinflammation. Annals of Neurology. 2015;**77**(5):784-803. DOI: 10.1002/ana.24380

[33] Liu S, Zhen G, Meloni BP, Campbell K, Winn HR. Rodent stroke model guidelines for preclinical stroke trials (1st edition). Journal of Experimental Stroke and Translational Medicine. 2009;**2**(2):2-27. DOI: 10.6030/1939-067X-2.2.2

[34] Dietrich WD, Ginsberg MD, Busto R, Watson BD. Photochemically induced cortical infarction in the rat. 1. Time course of hemodynamic consequences. Journal of Cerebral Blood Flow & Metabolism. 1986;**6**(2):184-194. DOI: 10.1038/jcbfm.1986.31

[35] Hossmann K-A. Cerebral ischemia: Models, methods and outcomes. Neuropharmacology. 2008;**55**(3): 257-270. DOI: 10.1016/j.neuropharm. 2007.12.004

[36] Wesley UV, Bhute VJ, Hatcher JF, Palecek SP, Dempsey RJ. Local and systemic metabolic alterations in brain, plasma, and liver of rats in response to aging and ischemic stroke, as detected by nuclear magnetic resonance (NMR) spectroscopy. Neurochemistry International. 2019;**127**:113-124. DOI: 10.1016/j.neuint.2019.01.025

[37] Nehlig A. Brain uptake and metabolism of ketone bodies in animal models. Prostaglandins, Leukotrienes and Essential Fatty Acids. 2004;**70**(3):265-275. DOI: 10.1016/j. plefa.2003.07.006

[38] Faria MHG, Muniz LRF, de Vasconcelos PRL. Ketone bodies metabolism during ischemic and reperfusion brain injuries following bilateral occlusion of common carotid arteries in rats. Acta Cirúrgica Brasileira. 2007;**22**(2):125-129. DOI: 10.1590/ S0102-86502007000200009

[39] Pinheiro PMA, Campelo APBS, Guimarães SB, do Patrocínio RMV, Junior JTV, de Vasconcelos PRL. Preconditioning with oil mixes of high ratio Omega-9: Omega-6 and a low ratio Omega-6:Omega-3 in rats subjected to brain ischemia/reperfusion. Acta Cirúrgica Brasileira. 2011;**26** (suppl. 1):32-37. DOI: 10.1590/ S0102-86502011000700007

[40] Campelo MWS et al. Preconditioning with a novel metallopharmaceutical NO donor in anesthetized rats subjected to brain ischemia/reperfusion. Neurochemical Research. 2012;**37**(4):749-758. DOI: 10.1007/s11064-011-0669-x

[41] Pires VL d S, de Souza JRF, Guimarães SB, Filho AR d S, Garcia JHP, de Vasconcelos PRL. Preconditioning with L-alanyl-L-glutamine in a Mongolian Gerbil model of acute cerebral ischemia/reperfusion injury. Acta Cirúrgica Brasileira. 2011;**26** (suppl 1):14-20. DOI: 10.1590/ S0102-86502011000700004

[42] de Oliveira LRA et al. Preconditioning with L-Ala-Gln reduces the expression of inflammatory markers (TNF-α, NF-κB, IL-6 and HO-1) in an injury animal model of cerebrovascular ischemia in Meriones unguiculatus (gerbils). Acta Cirúrgica Brasileira. 2020;**35**(6):1-9. DOI: 10.1590/ s0102-865020200060000001

[43] Vergouwen MDI et al. Definition of delayed cerebral ischemia after aneurysmal subarachnoid hemorrhage as an outcome event in clinical trials and observational studies. Stroke. 2010;**41**(10):2391-2395. DOI: 10.1161/ STROKEAHA.110.589275

[44] Foreman B. The pathophysiology of delayed cerebral ischemia. Journal of Clinical Neurophysiology. 2016;**33**(3):174-182. DOI: 10.1097/WNP.0000000000000273

[45] Hackenberg KAM, Hänggi D, Etminan N. Unruptured intracranial aneurysms. Stroke. 2018;**49**(9):2268-2275. DOI: 10.1161/STROKEAHA.118.021030

[46] Lucke-Wold B et al. Aneurysmal subarachnoid hemorrhage and neuroinflammation: A comprehensive review. International Journal of Molecular Sciences. 2016;**17**(4):1-17. DOI: 10.3390/ijms17040497

[47] Macdonald RL, Marton LS, Andrus PK, Hall ED, Johns L, Sajdak M. Time course of production of hydroxyl free radical after subarachnoid hemorrhage in dogs. Life Sciences. 2004;**75**(8):979-989. DOI: 10.1016/j.lfs.2004.02.010

[48] Chaichana KL, Pradilla G, Huang J, Tamargo RJ. Role of inflammation (leukocyte-endothelial cell interactions) in vasospasm after subarachnoid hemorrhage. World Neurosurgery. 2010;**73**(1):22-41. DOI: 10.1016/j.surneu.2009.05.027

[49] Gaastra B et al. CRP (C-Reactive Protein) in outcome prediction after subarachnoid hemorrhage and the role of machine learning. Stroke. 2021:3276-3285. DOI: 10.1161/STROKEAHA.120.030950

[50] Lee S, Kim YO, Ryu J-A. Clinical usefulness of early serial measurements of C-reactive protein as outcome predictors in patients with subarachnoid hemorrhage. BMC Neurology. 2020;**20**(1):1-10. DOI: 10.1186/s12883-020-01687-3

[51] Lucke-Wold B et al. Aneurysmal subarachnoid hemorrhage and neuroinflammation: A comprehensive review. International Journal of Molecular Sciences. 2016;**17**(4):1-17. DOI: 10.3390/ijms17040497

[52] Miller BA, Turan N, Chau M, Pradilla G. Inflammation, vasospasm, and brain injury after subarachnoid hemorrhage. BioMed Research International. 2014;**2014**:1-16. DOI: 10.1155/2014/384342

[53] Sarrafzadeh A, Schlenk F, Gericke C, Vajkoczy P. Relevance of cerebral interleukin-6 after aneurysmal subarachnoid hemorrhage. Neurocritical Care. 2010;**13**(3):339-346. DOI: 10.1007/s12028-010-9432-4

[54] Okada T, Suzuki H. Mechanisms of neuroinflammation and inflammatory mediators involved in brain injury following subarachnoid hemorrhage. Histology and Histopathology. 2020;**35**(7):623-636

[55] Villodre ES et al. NDRG1 expression is an independent prognostic factor in inflammatory breast cancer. Cancers. 2020;**12**(12):1-14. DOI: 10.3390/cancers12123711

[56] Qi B, Newcomer R, Sang Q-X. ADAM19/Adamalysin 19 structure, function, and role as a putative target in tumors and inflammatory diseases. Current Pharmaceutical Design. 2009;**15**(20):2336-2348. DOI: 10.2174/138161209788682352

[57] Santos JC, Bever SR, Pereira-da-Silva G, Pyter LM. Tumor resection ameliorates tumor-induced suppression of neuroinflammatory and behavioral responses to an immune challenge in a cancer survivor model. Scientific Reports. 2019;**9**(1):1-13. DOI: 10.1038/s41598-018-37334-8

[58] Sanchez-Perez Y, Soto-Reyes E, Garcia-Cuellar CM, Cacho-Diaz B, Santamaria A, Rangel-Lopez E. Role of epigenetics and oxidative stress in gliomagenesis. CNS & Neurological

Disorders - Drug Targets. 2018;**16**(10):1090-1098. DOI: 10.2174/1871527317666180110124645

[59] Sasaki A. Microglia and brain macrophages: An update. Neuropathology. 2017;**37**(5):452-464. DOI: 10.1111/neup.12354

[60] da Ros M et al. Glioblastoma chemoresistance: The double play by microenvironment and blood-brain barrier. International Journal of Molecular Sciences. 2018;**19**(10):1-23. DOI: 10.3390/ijms19102879

[61] Niklasson M et al. Mesenchymal transition and increased therapy resistance of glioblastoma cells is related to astrocyte reactivity. The Journal of Pathology. 2019;**249**(3):295-307. DOI: 10.1002/path.5317

[62] Lisi L, Stigliano E, Lauriola L, Navarra P, Dello Russo C. Proinflammatory-activated glioma cells induce a switch in microglial polarization and activation status, from a predominant M2b phenotype to a mixture of M1 and M2a/B polarized cells. ASN Neuro. 2014;**6**(3):171-183. DOI: 10.1042/AN20130045

[63] Ghoochani A et al. MIF-CD74 signaling impedes microglial M1 polarization and facilitates brain tumorigenesis. Oncogene. 2016;**35**(48):6246-6261. DOI: 10.1038/onc.2016.160

[64] Patri M, Singh A. Protective effects of noradrenaline on benzo[a]pyrene-induced oxidative stress responses in brain tumor cell lines. In Vitro Cellular & Developmental Biology. Animal. 2019;**55**(8):665-675. DOI: 10.1007/s11626-019-00378-9

[65] Maas SLN et al. Glioblastoma hijacks microglial gene expression to support tumor growth. Journal of Neuroinflammation. 2020;**17**(1):1-18. DOI: 10.1186/s12974-020-01797-2

[66] Yin Y, Qiu S, Li X, Huang B, Xu Y, Peng Y. EZH2 suppression in glioblastoma shifts microglia toward M1 phenotype in tumor microenvironment. Journal of Neuroinflammation. 2017;**14**(1):1-11. DOI: 10.1186/s12974-017-0993-4

[67] Sena IFG et al. Glioblastoma-activated pericytes support tumor growth via immunosuppression. Cancer Medicine. 2018;**7**(4):1232-1239. DOI: 10.1002/cam4.1375

[68] Qian J et al. The IFN-γ/PD-L1 axis between T cells and tumor microenvironment: Hints for glioma anti-PD-1/PD-L1 therapy. Journal of Neuroinflammation. 2018;**15**(1):1-13. DOI: 10.1186/s12974-018-1330-2

[69] Velayutham PK, Adhikary SD, Babu SK, Vedantam R, Korula G, Ramachandran A. Oxidative stress–associated hypertension in surgically induced brain injury patients: Effects of β-blocker and angiotensin-converting enzyme inhibitor. Journal of Surgical Research. 2013;**179**(1):125-131. DOI: 10.1016/j.jss.2012.09.005

[70] Dietrich WD, Chatzipanteli K, Vitarbo E, Wada K, Kinoshita K. The role of inflammatory processes in the pathophysiology and treatment of brain and spinal cord trauma. In: Mechanisms of Secondary Brain Damage from Trauma and Ischemia. Vienna: Springer Vienna; 2004. pp. 69-74. DOI: 10.1007/978-3-7091-0603-7_9

[71] Cerecedo-López CD, Kim-Lee JH, Hernandez D, Acosta SA, Borlongan CV. Insulin-associated neuroinflammatory pathways as therapeutic targets for traumatic brain injury. Medical Hypotheses. 2014;**82**(2):171-174. DOI: 10.1016/j.mehy.2013.11.028

[72] Kumar A et al. Microglial-derived microparticles mediate neuroinflammation after traumatic brain injury. Journal of

Neuroinflammation. 2017;**14**(1):1-17.
DOI: 10.1186/s12974-017-0819-4

[73] Younger D, Murugan M, Rao KVR, Wu L-J, Chandra N. Microglia receptors in animal models of traumatic brain injury. Molecular Neurobiology. 2019;**56**(7):5202-5228. DOI: 10.1007/s12035-018-1428-7

[74] Patel RK, Prasad N, Kuwar R, Haldar D, Abdul-Muneer PM. Transforming growth factor-beta 1 signaling regulates neuroinflammation and apoptosis in mild traumatic brain injury. Brain, Behavior, and Immunity. 2017;**64**:244-258. DOI: 10.1016/j.bbi.2017.04.012

[75] Kaplan GB et al. Pathophysiological bases of comorbidity: Traumatic brain injury and post-traumatic stress disorder. Journal of Neurotrauma. 2018;**35**(2):1-51. DOI: 10.1089/neu.2016.4953

[76] Miller MW, Lin AP, Wolf EJ, Miller DR. Oxidative stress, inflammation, and neuroprogression in chronic PTSD. Harvard Review of Psychiatry. 2018;**26**(2):57-69. DOI: 10.1097/HRP.0000000000000167

[77] Sulimai N, Lominadze D. Fibrinogen and Neuroinflammation During Traumatic Brain Injury. Molecular Neurobiology. 2020;**57**(11):4692-4703. DOI: 10.1007/s12035-020-02012-2

[78] Choi S et al. Regulation of endothelial barrier integrity by redox-dependent nitric oxide signaling: Implication in traumatic and inflammatory brain injuries. Nitric Oxide. 2019;**83**:51-64. DOI: 10.1016/j.niox.2018.12.007

[79] Abdul-Muneer PM, Chandra N, Haorah J. Interactions of oxidative stress and neurovascular inflammation in the pathogenesis of traumatic brain injury. Molecular Neurobiology.

2015;**51**(3):966-979. DOI: 10.1007/s12035-014-8752-3

[80] Borlongan C et al. Neuroinflammatory responses to traumatic brain injury: Etiology, clinical consequences, and therapeutic opportunities. Neuropsychiatric Disease and Treatment. 2015. pp. 97-106. DOI: 10.2147/NDT.S65815

[81] Stamatovic SM, Dimitrijevic OB, Keep RF, Andjelkovic AV. Inflammation and brain edema: New insights into the role of chemokines and their receptors. In: Brain Edema XIII. Vienna: Springer-Verlag. pp. 444-450. DOI: 10.1007/3-211-30714-1_91

Chapter 2

Cerebrovascular Disease and Hypertension

Navdeep Singh Sidhu and Sumandeep Kaur

Abstract

Systemic hypertension is a major public health problem, nearly affecting one-third of the global adult population. It is the leading modifiable risk factor for coronary heart disease (CHD), cerebrovascular disease, renal dysfunction, peripheral arterial disease (PAD), heart failure and atrial fibrillation. Human brain is one of the most important target organs for hypertension related end-organ damage. Two major categories of hypertension related cerebral diseases include stroke and dementia, which are associated with considerable morbidity and mortality. Large body of clinical evidence has shown that adequate control of elevated blood pressures (BPs) could be a very effective tool in reducing the incidence and prevalence of cerebrovascular diseases. In the following sections, we discuss the role of hypertension in the causation of cerebrovascular disease along with the preventive and therapeutic strategies for the same.

Keywords: cerebrovascular disease, stroke, dementia, blood pressure, hypertension, intracranial hemorrhage, management, brain, cerebral, ischemic

1. Introduction

Systemic hypertension is one of the most common and devastating disorders affecting the human race. It is a major cause of premature death worldwide and is the risk factor with greatest impact on the global burden of disease. It is the leading modifiable risk factor for cardiovascular disease and all-cause mortality [1, 2].

Worldwide, an estimated 1.38 billion individuals (31.1% of the adult population) have hypertension, defined as systolic blood pressure (BP) ≥ 140 mm Hg and/or diastolic BP ≥ 90 mm Hg, and/or current use of antihypertensive medication. The age-standardized prevalence of hypertension is marginally higher in men (31.9%) than in women (30.1%) and is lower in high-income countries (HICs), as compared to low and middle-income countries (LMICs) (28.5% vs. 31.5%) [3]. According to global estimates in 2010, only 45.6% of individuals with hypertension were aware of the disease, only 36.9% were receiving treatment and only 13.8% had achieved adequate BP control (defined as systolic BP < 140 mm Hg and diastolic BP < 90 mm Hg). Also, the proportion of hypertension awareness and treatment was nearly twice and the proportion of hypertension control was four times in HICs as compared to LMICs. In the last 2 decades, HICs have shown substantial increases in the proportions of hypertension awareness, treatment and control. However, during the same period, awareness and treatment have increased only modestly in LMICs and the proportion of hypertensive patients having adequately controlled BP has decreased slightly [3].

The global prevalence of hypertension is increasing steadily as a result of aging of the population and increase in lifestyle risk factors like unhealthy diets (high sodium, low potassium intake, high intake of saturated and trans-fats and low intake of fruits and vegetables), physical inactivity, increased consumption of alcohol and tobacco, and being overweight or obese. However, the changes in the prevalence of hypertension have not been uniform worldwide. In the last two decades, a modest decline has been noted in hypertension prevalence in HICs, whereas LMICs have experienced significant increases. These trends can impose a greater burden of hypertension and related cardiovascular disorders on the fragile health-care systems of LMICs, many of which are also facing a substantial burden of infectious diseases [4].

Hypertension is often called a "silent killer", as most hypertensives are unaware of the problem due to lack of warning symptoms or signs. Hypertension can cause sub-clinical target organ damage for years, before any symptoms or signs develop. It is the leading modifiable risk factor implicated in the causation of coronary heart disease (CHD), cerebrovascular disease, renal dysfunction, peripheral arterial disease (PAD), heart failure and atrial fibrillation. The brain is a major target for hypertension related end-organ damage and hypertension is a prominent risk factor for two major categories of brain diseases: stroke and dementia. In the following sections, we discuss the role of hypertension in causation of these diseases, along with prevention and treatment strategies.

2. Hypertension and brain

Human brain, in general, is highly vulnerable to the harmful effects of elevated BP and it represents the classic target organ of hypertension-induced damage. Arterial hypertension, besides being responsible for its well-known effect in causing clinical stroke, is also associated with the development of asymptomatic, subclinical brain damage, such as cerebral small vessel disease with resultant cognitive impairment, memory loss and dementia. Also, sudden and marked elevations of blood pressure can lead to the development of hypertensive encephalopathy, characterized by severe headache, seizures and other neurological symptoms like cerebral edema.

2.1 Hypertension and stroke

2.1.1 Hypertension as a risk factor for stroke

Globally, stroke ranks second among the causes of mortality and third among the causes of disability. In recent decades a trend towards reduction in the incidence, prevalence and mortality of stroke has been noted, but the overall disease burden continues to rise in terms of total number of patients affected [5].

Stroke is usually categorized into ischemic and hemorrhagic forms. Ischemic stroke has further subtypes including large vessel occlusive disease, lacunar infarctions due to small vessel disease, cerebral embolism including cardioembolic stroke, non-atherogenic stroke and cryptogenic stroke. Various subtypes of hemorrhagic stroke include intra-parenchymal hemorrhage, subarachnoid hemorrhage and intraventricular hemorrhage.

Hypertension is the most prevalent risk factor for stroke and has been reported in nearly two-thirds of stroke patients [6]. In LMICs, the reported prevalence of risk factors among patients with stroke is lower, however the in-hospital mortality rates have been higher, probably related to delays in presentation, differences in healthcare system responses and acute management of stroke [7].

There is robust evidence from observational and interventional studies, implicating hypertension as a strong risk factor for all types of strokes. The Framingham heart study in 1970 showed a significant association between the risk of stroke and blood pressure ≥ 160/95 mm Hg at all ages and in both sexes [8]. Persons with a normal BP (<120/80 mm Hg) had been reported approximately half the lifetime risk of stroke compared to those with high BP (≥140/90 mm Hg) [9].

Large epidemiological studies have consistently shown the relationship between the level of BP and risk of stroke to be consistent, continuous, and independent of other risk factors. Older epidemiological studies gave more importance to the diastolic BP as a determinant of stroke risk, and consistently showed a higher risk of stroke with increasing levels of diastolic BP [10, 11]. MacMahon et al., in their meta-analysis of nine observational studies conducted between 1958 and 1990, showed that as the level of BP decreased so did the risk of stroke. A decrease in diastolic BP of 5, 7.5, and 10 mm Hg was associated with a lowering of stroke risk by 34, 46, and 56%, respectively [11]. Similarly, The Eastern Stroke and Coronary Heart Disease Collaborative Research project, showed that for every 5 mm Hg fall in the diastolic BP resulted in nearly 50% reduction in the risk of ischemic (odds ratio (OR) 0.61; 95% confidence interval 0.57–0.66) and hemorrhagic stroke (odds ratio 0.54, 95% confidence interval 0.50–0.58) [12]. Systolic BP attracted greater attention in 1990s after the results from many epidemiological studies suggested that it could have more robust association with stroke as compared to diastolic BP. Systolic BP also showed a stronger correlation with 12 year stroke mortality than the diastolic BP in Framingham heart study [13]. Similarly, the prospective population-based Copenhagen city heart study demonstrated systolic BP to be a better predictor of stroke than the diastolic BP [14]. The Asia Pacific Cohort Studies Collaboration (APCSC), an extension of the Eastern Stroke and Coronary Heart Disease Collaborative project, which analyzed 37 cohort studies of 425,325 patients in the Asia Pacific region, demonstrated a continuous, log-linear association between systolic BP and risk of stroke down to the levels of 115 mm Hg of systolic BP. In the age groups of <60, 60–69, and >70 years, a 10 mm Hg lower systolic BP was associated with 54%, 36% and 25% lower risk of stroke respectively [15]. In a meta-analysis of 61 prospective studies by the Prospective Study Collaboration (PSC), it was demonstrated that there was more than a twofold decrease in stroke mortality with each 20 mm Hg of decrease in systolic BP for patients aged 40–69 years; and throughout middle and old age, usual BP is directly and strongly related to vascular (and overall) mortality, without any evidence of a threshold down to at least 115 mm Hg of systolic BP and 75 mm Hg of diastolic BP [16].

Age is an important cofactor in the relationship between hypertension and stroke. The direct relation between elevated BP and stroke risk is weaker in older aged populations than in middle-aged individuals. The APCSC observed a lower percentage reduction in stroke risk with similar reduction in systolic BP with increasing age [15]. A similar trend was observed in the PSC study [16]. Although there is a less robust association between hypertension and stroke risk in older populations, lowering BP in this population is still beneficial owing to the higher incidence of stroke and higher morbidity/mortality rates in this population [17].

Racial and ethnic disparities in the relationship between elevated BP and stroke have been reported from several observational studies from the United States. The Baltimore-Washington Cooperative Young Stroke Study, demonstrated a positive relationship between hypertension and the risk of ischemic stroke in whites and blacks for both sexes. In this study, age-adjusted odds ratios and 95% confidence interval for ischemic stroke with a history of hypertension in white males, white females, black males, and black females were 1.6 (0.7–3.2), 2.5 (1.1–5.9), 3.8 (1.8–7.9), and 4.2 (2.4–7.5), respectively [18]. Similarly, the Northern Manhattan Stroke

Study showed higher odds ratios for hypertension and ischemic stroke in blacks as compared to whites and hispanics (OR 2.0 vs. 1.8, 1.2 respectively) [19]. A similar increase in systolic BP is associated with a nearly three times higher risk of stroke risk in blacks as compared to whites [20].

2.1.2 Hypertension related stroke and its pathophysiological mechanisms

Although arterial hypertension is a major risk factor for both stroke and myocardial infarction, stroke is much more closely related to elevated levels of BP per se. It has been suggested that a sustained reduction in systolic blood pressure of 10 mm Hg would reduce stroke risk by 56%, but reduce the risk of myocardial infarction by only 37% [11]. This difference is largely attributed to the possibility that elevated levels of blood pressure are directly responsible for strokes occurring due to small vessel disease, but is only indirectly related to the development of atherosclerotic changes. Atherosclerosis in the arterial tree is usually focal and is usually seen at the branching points of the arteries or where arteries take a bend. It is likely that the effects of hypertension on atherosclerosis are not per se due to pressure energy, but are more likely related to the transmission of kinetic energy to the arterial wall at sites of flow disturbance, thus leading to the formation of atherosclerotic plaques at the areas of low shear stress [21].

Strokes due to small vessel disease, in contrast, are directly caused by elevated blood pressure. For this reason, these tend to occur in a particular distribution at the base of the brain, where short, straight arteries with limited branches result in direct transmission of high blood pressure directly from the large arteries to the smaller resistance vessels, with resultant damage to the walls of the arterioles. This results in the pathological changes of hyaline degeneration and fibrinoid necrosis, with consequent lacunar infarctions where the arterioles occlude and hypertensive intracerebral hemorrhages where they rupture. These pathophysiological changes account for the fact that true lacunar infarctions and intracerebral hemorrhages are particularly distributed in the areas of basal ganglia, internal capsule, thalamus, cerebellum, and brainstem [22].

Hypertension can indirectly contribute to the development of stroke as it is an important etiological factor for atrial fibrillation and for acute myocardial infarction and left ventricular clot formation; with attendant risk of cardioembolic stroke.

There are many theories related to the pathophysiological mechanisms of hypertension related brain dysfunction. Central to these theories are the mechanisms related to impaired cerebrovascular auto-regulation in hypertension and the chronic maladaptive changes in the structure of the cerebral vasculature in hypertensive patients.

Cerebrovascular autoregulation is the process by which cerebral vasculature regulates intracranial blood flow, so that a steady perfusion is maintained to meet the metabolic needs of the brain tissue across a range of systemic blood pressures. This control is achieved by the ability of the cerebral arterioles to compensate for a decrease in cerebral perfusion pressure by vasodilatation, and also, to protect the brain against increased perfusion pressure by vasoconstriction, thus keeping the cerebral blood flow constant. This complex process is regulated by interplay between sympathetic nervous system, brain carbon dioxide and other metabolites, and neurovascular coupling. In normotensive individuals, this response occurs over a range of approximately 60–160 mm Hg systolic BP; but, in patients with hypertension, this range may be shifted to higher pressures [23, 24]. This upward shift in the limits of pressure autoregulation, make hypertensive patients especially susceptible to episodes of hypotension, which plays a role in the development of white matter changes. Also, elderly hypertensive patients often have impaired cerebrovascular autoregulation which contributes to the development of stroke, cognitive dysfunction and vascular dementia. Impaired autoregulation increases the transmission of elevated pressures to cerebral capillaries resulting in increased permeability of blood brain barrier (BBB), parenchymal edema, inflammation neuronal degeneration that is commonly seen in patients with vascular cognitive dysfunction [25]. Chronic hypertension has been reported to promote arteriolar and capillary rarefaction, especially in the deep hemispherical white matter and basal ganglia [26]. This is associated with infiltration of perivascular macrophages, endothelial dysfunction, increased oxidative stress, and impaired functional hyperemia [27]. These changes promote the development of lacunar infarcts, white matter hyper-intensities, microinfarcts, and microbleeds [28].

Chronic elevation of intraluminal pressure stimulates the growth of smooth muscle cells and increases media thickness in resistance arteries, resulting in hypertrophic remodeling, thus causing an elevated vascular resistance. There may also be eutrophic remodeling, characterized by inward remodeling with rearrangement of the vessel wall components that leads to a reduction in lumen diameter and elevated vascular resistance. Hypertension may also result in narrowing of the intermediate and small vessels due to lipo-hyalinosis and micro-atherosclerosis. Also, chronically elevated BP promotes hyaline degeneration, fibrinoid degeneration and formation of microaneurysms in small vessels of the cerebral vasculature. These small vessel alterations predispose these patients to the development of ischemic and hemorrhagic complications [29].

Hypertension promotes atherosclerosis in large extracranial and intracranial arteries, which predispose to the development of atherothrombotic infarctions. The most frequent sites of atherosclerosis are common carotid artery bifurcation, origin and intra-cavernous part of internal carotid artery, first segment of middle cerebral artery, origin and distal part of vertebral artery, and middle portion of basilar artery [29]. These atherosclerotic plaques are usually progressive and lead to ischemic strokes by thrombotic occlusion of the narrowed lumen or, more often, by their acute rupture, which causes atheroembolism resulting in occlusion of distal intracranial vessels [29]. Major mechanisms of hypertension related cerebral dysfunction are summarized in **Table 1**.

2.1.3 Blood pressure management for primary and secondary stroke prevention

2.1.3.1 Hypertension control for primary stroke prevention

The relation between BP and stroke risk is direct, strong, linear, and etiologically predictive. Thus, within the usual BP ranges, including non-hypertensive ones, the higher levels of BP are associated with increased risk of stroke [16]. Non-hypertensive individuals with slight elevations of BP (prehypertension, defined as systolic BP of 120–139 mm Hg and/or diastolic BP of 80–89 mm Hg) derive benefit

Impairment of cerebral autoregulation
Increased permeability of blood brain barrier
Endothelial dysfunction, oxidative stress, impaired functional hyperemia
Small vessel changes: remodeling, increased vascular resistance, lipo-hyalinosis, micro-atherosclerosis, micro aneurysms, lacunar infarcts
Large vessel changes: atherosclerosis with atherothrombotic, atheroembolic infarctions

Table 1.
Potential mechanisms of hypertension related cerebral dysfunction.

from lifestyle changes with or without pharmacological therapies. A meta-analysis with 70,664 prehypertensive individuals from 16 trials demonstrated a robust 22% reduction in the stroke risk in individuals randomized to pharmacological therapy arm as compared to the placebo arm. In hypertensive patients, lifestyle approaches combined with adequate BP treatment and control produced a 35–40% decrease in the stroke risk [30, 31].

Practical strategies for hypertension management for primary stroke prevention, on the basis of recommendations made by the American Heart Association (AHA)/American Stroke Association (ASA) [32, 33], and European Society of Cardiology (ESC)/European Society of Hypertension (ESH) [34] include:

1. Regular screening for hypertension and management of raised BP using lifestyle modifications and pharmacological therapies are recommended.

2. According to European guidelines the target BP in those with hypertension should be <140/90 mm Hg, whereas, the recent American guidelines recommend a BP goal to lower levels of <130/80 mm Hg, even in very elderly.

3. Successful attainment of BP goal is emphasized over the administration of a particular anti-hypertensive agent.

4. Individualized BP treatment is recommended, based on particular patient characteristics and tolerance to medications.

5. Self-monitoring of BP is recommended to help in adequate BP control.

2.1.3.2 Hypertension management in acute ischemic stroke

Management of elevated BP in acute ischemic stroke (AIS) has been a matter of considerable debate. AIS is usually associated with islands of infarcted tissue with surrounding areas of potentially salvageable tissue, referred to as ischemic penumbra. Moreover, the infarcted tissue is characterized by loss of autoregulation with increased vessel permeability [35]. Hence an over aggressive approach of lowering BP can result in extension of infarction and worsening of neurological dysfunction. On the other hand, if the elevated BP is not lowered sufficiently, there is risk of excessive cerebral edema and hemorrhagic transformation of the infarcted tissue. Furthermore, as the cerebrovascular auto regulatory response is set at a higher level in chronic hypertensive patients, these individuals are at risk of impaired cerebral perfusion if BP is lowered very aggressively.

Practical strategies for management of hypertension in AIS, based on recommendations of AHA/ASA [36], and European stroke organization (ESO) [37] include:

1. In patients with AIS who are not eligible for systemic thrombolysis or mechanical thrombectomy and who have a BP > 220/120 mm Hg, guarded BP reduction (<15% systolic BP reduction over 24 h) is reasonable and is likely to be safe. No recommendations are made regarding the use of a specific anti-hypertensive agent to achieve this goal.

2. In hospitalized patients with AIS and blood pressure < 220/110 mm Hg not treated with intravenous thrombolysis or mechanical thrombectomy, there is suggestion against the routine use of blood pressure lowering agents at least in first 24 h following symptom onset, unless this is necessary for specific comorbid

conditions like acute aortic dissection, acute myocardial infarction, pulmonary edema, hypertensive encephalopathy and acute renal failure.

3. In patients with AIS undergoing treatment with intravenous thrombolysis (with or without mechanical thrombectomy) it is suggested that BP is maintained below 185/110 mm Hg before bolus and below 180/105 mm Hg after bolus, and for 24 h after alteplase infusion.

4. In patients with AIS undergoing treatment with intravenous thrombolysis (with or without mechanical thrombectomy), there is suggestion against lowering systolic blood pressure to a target of 130–140 mm Hg compared to <180 mm Hg during the first 72 h following of symptom onset.

5. Initiating or continuing anti-hypertensive agents during hospitalization for AIS, if BP > 140/90 mm Hg: BP lowering is generally safe in AIS if patient is medically and neurologically stable, and there are no contraindications for BP lowering. The time window for administration of such therapies is usually 2–3 days after the symptom onset.

Drug options to treat hypertension in patients with AIS who are planned for emergency reperfusion therapy are shown in **Table 2**.

2.1.3.3 Hypertension management in acute hemorrhagic stroke

Observational studies have suggested that BP is often markedly elevated in the acute phase of hemorrhagic stroke, significantly higher than that seen after AIS [38]. High levels of BP in acute hemorrhagic stroke are often associated with hematoma expansion and poor clinical outcomes [39]. Simultaneously, there have been suggestions that high BP may be necessary to maintain adequate cerebral perfusion after intracranial hemorrhage, and that aggressively lowering it may be deleterious. These concerns are however, opposed by the evidence suggesting that adequate cerebral perfusion is maintained after acute BP reduction in patients with hemorrhagic stroke [40, 41]. However, results of the two largest randomized clinical trials (INTERACT2, ATACH-2) of intensive BP lowering early after intracranial hemorrhage have renewed this uncertainty [42, 43]. Meta-analyses of these trials and many other smaller studies have shown that early intensive BP reduction after hemorrhagic stroke is safe, but without mortality benefit or significant functional improvement [44–47]. In contrast, a recent meta-analysis of the two largest trials demonstrated a direct linear relation between the level of systolic BP

Labetalol: 10–20 mg intra-venous over 1–2 min, may be repeated once; or
Nicardipine: 5 mg/h intra-venous, dose may be up-titrated by 2.5 mg/h in every 5–15 min to a maximum of 15 mg/h; when desired BP levels is obtained, adjust the dose to maintain proper BP levels; or
Clevidipine: 1–2 mg/h intra-venous, up-titrate by doubling the dose in every 2–5 min until desired BP level is obtained; maximum dose 21 mg/h
Other agents like enalaprilat, hydralazine may also be useful
If BP is not controlled or diastolic BP > 140 mm Hg, consider intravenous nitroprusside (may increase intracranial pressure).

Table 2.
Drugs for acute management of elevated blood pressures in patients of acute ischemic stroke who are planned for emergency reperfusion therapy [36, 37].

achieved during the first 24 h of hemorrhagic stroke and the functional status. The improvements in the functional status were noted for systolic BP levels of as low as 120–130 mm Hg [48]. These studies however excluded patients with severe, large hematomas and hence caution is warranted in too aggressive lowering of BP in such patients as it might predispose to harmful consequences [49].

Practical strategies for BP control in patients with acute hemorrhagic stroke based on recent AHA/ASA [50], and ESO [37] guidelines include:

1. If initial systolic BP is >220 mm Hg, it is reasonable to administer continuous intravenous BP lowering therapy to achieve an initial reduction of about 15%. Choice of drugs is similar to that used in AIS (**Table 2**).

2. In patients with initial systolic BP of 150–220 mm Hg, American guidelines suggest a target goal of 140–150 mm Hg of systolic BP [50], however, the recent ESO guidelines [37] recommend even more aggressive lowering of systolic BP to less than 140 mm Hg (but to keep it above 110 mm Hg) to reduce hepatoma expansion.

3. Control of blood pressure variability may be helpful in improving the outcomes [51].

4. After hemorrhagic stroke, the optimal timing for initiation of antihypertensive therapies for secondary stroke prevention has not been well established. It may be reasonable to start such treatment when the patient is medically and neurologically stable. The target BP goal for secondary stroke prevention is <130/80 mm Hg [50].

2.1.3.4 Hypertension management for secondary stroke prevention

About a quarter of strokes are recurrent, the annual risk of recurrence is nearly 4% and the mortality rate after a recurrent stroke is 41% [33, 34]. A large proportion of strokes can be prevented by adequate BP control, regular physical activity, healthy dietary habits and cessation of smoking. In fact, the INTERSTROKE study demonstrated that these 5 factors—hypertension, imbalanced diet, lack of adequate physical activity, abdominal obesity and smoking—were responsible for 82% and 90% of the population attributable risk (PAR) for ischemic and hemorrhagic stroke respectively [6]. Also, the Global Burden of Disease Study suggested that nearly 90% of the global stroke burden was attributable to the modifiable risk factors [52]. A modeling study has shown that targeting multiple modifiable risk factors of stroke has additive benefits in secondary prevention of stroke. According to this study, aspirin, anti-hypertensive therapies and statins, along with dietary modification and adequate exercise, can lead to an 80% cumulative risk reduction in the incidence of recurrent vascular events [53].

Practical strategies for BP control for secondary recent AHA/ASA guidelines [54] include:

1. In hypertensive patients who suffer a stroke or transient ischemic attack (TIA), an office BP goal of <130/80 mm Hg is recommended for most patients to reduce the risk of recurrent stroke and vascular events.

2. In individuals with no history of hypertension who experience a stroke or TIA and have an average office BP of ≥130/80 mm Hg, antihypertensive drug treatment can be beneficial to decrease the risk of recurrent stroke, intracranial hemorrhage, and other vascular events.

3. A thiazide diuretic, angiotensin converting enzyme (ACE) inhibitor or angiotensin receptor blocker (ARB) may be useful, however, other classes of BP lowering therapy can be used to achieve the target BP goals (e.g., calcium channel blocker, newer generation beta blocker).

4. Individualized drug treatments that take into account patient comorbidities, pharmacological class of the drug, and patient preferences are recommended to maximize the drug efficacy.

2.2 Hypertension and dementia

2.2.1 Hypertension as a risk factor for cognitive dysfunction and dementia

Dementia is characterized by a progressive and often irreversible decline of cognitive function which is most commonly seen in older adults. It is one of the most common neurological diseases, nearly affecting 30–40 million people worldwide. The number of people with dementia is estimated to triple by 2050, largely driven by the aging of the population, demographic shifts, and lack of disease-modifying therapies [55]. Alzheimer disease (AD) and cerebrovascular diseases are the major causes of cognitive dysfunction, accounting for nearly 80% of the cases and often have a mixture of both the pathologies [55]. Although the majority of dementias including AD are primarily considered as neuro-degenerative diseases of unknown cause, recent studies have shown that cerebrovascular disease and microscopic vascular lesions are often found in patients affected by these conditions [56].

The term vascular cognitive impairment (VCI) refers to the entire spectrum of cognitive abnormalities caused by vascular etiologies, whereas the term vascular dementia is used for cases with more profound vascular cognitive deficits which negatively affect the daily functioning of an individual [57].

Among the various vascular risk factors, systemic hypertension is a major factor contributing to cognitive impairment [57]. It has been been associated with decreased abstract reasoning, reduced mental processing speed, and, less commonly, memory deficits [58]. Although dementia due to AD and vascular dementia have classically been considered as separate entities, recent evidence indicates that the two conditions are frequently coexistent [59, 60]. In nearly 40–50% of cases with a clinical diagnosis of AD, the pathological hallmarks of AD (amyloid plaques and the neurofibrillary tangles), are associated with micro-cerebrovascular and macro-cerebrovascular lesions [61]. Moreover, ischemic lesions markedly elevate the effect of AD pathology on cognitive function [62, 63]. Also, traditional cardiovascular risk factors have been suggested to have a role in the development of AD [64], and some estimates suggest that risk factor modification, especially the treatment of hypertension, could decrease the incidence of clinically diagnosed AD by up-to 30% [65].

2.2.2 Mechanisms of hypertension related cognitive dysfunction

Hypertension-related cognitive dysfunction occurs as a result of complex interplay between functional alterations and structural changes seen in the brain parenchyma and the cerebral vasculature, many of which have been discussed previously in Section 2.1.2. Briefly, these changes include increased cerebrovascular resistance, reduced vasomotor reactivity, decreased cerebral blood flow, vascular remodeling, lacunar infarcts, white matter lesions, micro bleeds, enlarged perivascular spaces and cerebral atrophy [66]. These overlapping pathophysiological changes might account for the correlation between hypertension and stroke or vascular dementia.

This relation may also hold true for other forms of dementia; like, for example the link between chronic hypertension and the AD has been documented, as hypertension is often associated with formation of neurofibrillary tangles and senile plaques, the presence of which was seen in brains of hypertensive patients even in the absence of clinical features of dementia [67].

2.2.3 Prevention of cognitive dysfunction by antihypertensive therapy

Hypertension is a major modifiable risk factor for cognitive dysfunction, VCI and AD. Robust clinical evidence has demonstrated that antihypertensive therapies, besides preventing major cerebrovascular events [57], also reduce the incidence and/or delay the progression of cognitive dysfunction [68, 69]. The Syst-Eur randomized clinical trial showed that, on treating 1000 hypertensive individuals with anti-hypertension therapies for 5 years, 19 cases of dementia could be prevented [70]. Similarly, the PROGRESS trial observed that therapy with a perindopril (a long-acting ACE inhibitor), and indapamide (a thiazide-like diuretic), was associated with reduced risks of cognitive dysfunction and dementia on a mean follow-up of 3.9 years [71]. Also, various clinical and experimental studies have suggested that antihypertensive drugs, including ACE inhibitors, angiotensin receptor blockers (ARBs) and diuretics, might cause an improvement in the biomarkers of AD, and decrease the incidence of AD and/or delay its progression [72].

Interestingly, antihypertensive drug therapies might have class specific effects on cognitive function. Both ACE inhibitors and calcium channel blockers have been reported to delay the development of cognitive dysfunction [72]. However, results from the Canadian Study of Health and Aging suggested that hypertensive individuals aged ≥65 years who received treatment with calcium channel blockers had a more marked cognitive decline than those receiving other antihypertensive drugs at follow-up of 5 years [73]. These findings lend support to the hypothesis that the systemic and local renin-angiotensin systems may respond differently to different antihypertensive drugs [74]. Furthermore, calcium channel blockers may potentially cause an impairment of myogenic autoregulatory protective responses in the cerebral vasculature. Taking these factors into account, it might be suggested that ACE inhibitors and ARBs might be preferable to calcium channel antagonists for dementia prevention in hypertensive patients [75].

The subject of optimum BP targets for the prevention of dementia has generated considerable debate and controversy. In the SPRINT MIND trial, it was seen that in ambulatory hypertensive individuals, a more intensive BP control strategy (target systolic BP of <120 mm Hg as compared to a target of <140 mm Hg) was not associated with any significant cognitive benefits [76]. An important point to be considered here is that due to the adaptive rightward shift of the cerebrovascular autoregulatory curve in hypertension, too aggressive lowering of BP may result in cerebral hypoperfusion and consequential negative impact on the brain. These U-shaped associations between BP and cognitive function in the elderly individuals have been reported in many studies [77, 78]. These findings stress the importance of individualized blood pressure management strategies for prevention of cognitive dysfunction.

Hypertension is also a major contributor to the risk of stroke, which nearly doubles the risk of developing dementia. It is estimated that about one-third cases of dementia can be prevented by preventing the development of stroke [79]. Clinical studies have shown that prevention of stroke by using anticoagulation in atrial fibrillation and BP-lowering therapies in hypertensive patients can significantly decrease the risk of dementia [80]. Based on these results, the World Stroke Organization came out with a manifesto stressing the need for a joint strategy for prevention of stroke and dementia [79].

3. Conclusions

Hypertension is a major global public health problem and is the major cause of premature death worldwide. Human brain is highly vulnerable to the deleterious effects of elevated blood pressures. Hypertension related cerebrovascular diseases include stroke, cognitive dysfunction and dementia. Elevated blood pressure levels are strongly, directly and linearly related to the incidence and prevalence of these diseases. Adequate management of hypertension can go a long way in mitigating the global burden of these cerebrovascular diseases.

4. Final remarks

Elevated systemic blood pressures are associated with increased risk of cerebrovascular diseases including stroke and dementia. Good blood pressure control, which can be achieved easily in majority of the patients, is necessary for prevention of these cerebrovascular diseases.

Author details

Navdeep Singh Sidhu[1*] and Sumandeep Kaur[2]

1 Department of Cardiology, GGS Medical College and Baba Farid University of Health Sciences, Faridkot, Punjab, India

2 Faculty of Nursing Sciences, Baba Farid University of Health Sciences, Faridkot, Punjab, India

*Address all correspondence to: navsids@gmail.com

IntechOpen

References

[1] GBD 2017 Causes of Death Collaborators. Global, regional, and national age-sex-specific mortality for 282 causes of death in 195 countries and territories, 1980-2017: A systematic analysis for the global burden of disease study 2017. The Lancet. 2018; 392(10159):1736-1788. DOI: 10.1016/S0140-6736(18)32203-7

[2] GBD 2017 Risk Factor Collaborators. Global, regional, and national comparative risk assessment of 84 behavioural, environmental and occupational, and metabolic risks or clusters of risks for 195 countries and territories, 1990-2017: A systematic analysis for the global burden of disease study 2017. The Lancet. 2018; 10, 392(10159):1923-1994. DOI: 10.1016/S0140-6736(18)32225-6

[3] Mills KT, Bundy JD, Kelly TN, Reed JE, Kearney PM, Reynolds K, et al. Global disparities of hypertension prevalence and control: A systematic analysis of population-based studies from 90 countries. Circulation. 2016; 134(6):441-450. DOI: 10.1161/CIRCULATIONAHA.115.018912

[4] NCD Risk Factor Collaboration (NCD-RisC). Worldwide trends in blood pressure from 1975 to 2015: A pooled analysis of 1479 population-based measurement studies with 19·1 million participants. The Lancet. 2017;389(10064):37-55. DOI: 10.1016/S0140-6736(16)31919-5

[5] Feigin VL, Norrving B, Mensah GA. Global burden of stroke. Circulation Research. 2017;120(3):439-448. DOI: 10.1161/CIRCRESAHA.116.308413

[6] O'Donnell MJ, Xavier D, Liu L, Zhang H, Chin SL, Rao-Melacini P, et al. Risk factors for ischaemic and intracerebral haemorrhagic stroke in 22 countries (the INTERSTROKE study): A case-control study. The Lancet. 2010;376(9735):112-123. DOI: 10.1016/S0140-6736(10)60834-3

[7] Khatib R, Arevalo YA, Berendsen MA, Prabhakaran S, Huffman MD. Presentation, evaluation, management, and outcomes of acute stroke in low- and middle-income countries: A systematic review and meta-analysis. Neuroepidemiology. 2018;51(1-2):104-112. DOI: 10.1159/000491442

[8] Kannel WB, Wolf PA, Verter J, McNamara PM. Epidemiologic assessment of the role of blood pressure in stroke. The Framingham study. Journal of the American Medical Association. 1970;214:301-310

[9] Seshadri S, Beiser A, Kelly-Hayes M, Kase CS, Au R, Kannel WB, et al. The lifetime risk of stroke: Estimates from the Framingham Study. Stroke. 2006; 37:345-350

[10] Prospective Studies Collaboration. Cholesterol, diastolic blood pressure, and stroke: 13,000 strokes in 450,000 people in 45 prospective cohorts. The Lancet. 1995;346:1647-1653

[11] MacMahon S, Peto R, Cutler J, Collins R, Sorlie P, Neaton J, et al. Blood pressure, stroke, and coronary heart disease. Part 1, prolonged differences in blood pressure: Prospective observational studies corrected for the regression dilution bias. The Lancet. 1990;335:765-774

[12] Eastern Stroke and Coronary Heart Disease Collaborative Research Group. Blood pressure, cholesterol, and stroke in eastern Asia. The Lancet. 1998; 352:1801-1807

[13] Kannel WB, Wolf PA, McGee DL, Dawber TR, McNamara P, Castelli WP. Systolic blood pressure, arterial rigidity, and risk of stroke. The Framingham

study. Journal of the American Medical Association. 1981;**245**:1225-1229

[14] Nielsen WB, Lindenstrom E, Vestbo J, Jensen GB. Is diastolic hypertension an independent risk factor for stroke in the presence of normal systolic blood pressure in the middle-aged and elderly? American Journal of Hypertension. 1997;**10**:634-639

[15] Lawes CM, Rodgers A, Bennett DA, Parag V, Suh I, Ueshima H, et al. Blood pressure and cardiovascular disease in the Asia Pacific region. Journal of Hypertension. 2003;**21**:707-716

[16] Lewington S, Clarke R, Qizilbash N, Peto R, Collins R. Prospective Studies Collaboration. Age-specific relevance of usual blood pressure to vascular mortality: A meta-analysis of individual data for one million adults in 61 prospective studies. The Lancet. 2002;**360**(9349):1903-1913. DOI: 10.1016/s0140-6736(02)11911-8

[17] Lawes CM, Bennett DA, Feigin VL, Rodgers A. Blood pressure and stroke: an overview of published reviews. Stroke. 2004;**35**:776-785

[18] Rohr J, Kittner S, Feeser B, Hebel JR, Whyte MG, Weinstein A, et al. Traditional risk factors and ischemic stroke in young adults: The Baltimore-Washington Cooperative Young Stroke Study. Archives of Neurology. 1996; **53**:603-607

[19] Sacco RL, Boden-Albala B, Abel G, Lin IF, Elkind M, Hauser WA, et al. Race-ethnic disparities in the impact of stroke risk factors: The northern Manhattan stroke study. Stroke. 2001; **32**:1725-1731

[20] Howard G, Lackland DT, Kleindorfer DO, Kissela BM, Moy CS, Judd SE, et al. Racial differences in the impact of elevated systolic blood pressure on stroke risk. JAMA Internal Medicine. 2013;**173**:46-51

[21] Spence JD. Effects of antihypertensive agents on blood velocity: Implications for atherogenesis. Canadian Medical Association Journal. 1982;**127**(8):721-724

[22] Soros P, Whitehead S, Spence JD, Hachinski V. Antihypertensive treatment can prevent stroke and cognitive decline. Nature Reviews Neurology. 2013;**9**(3):174-178

[23] Paulson OB, Strandgaard S, Fau-Edvinsson L, Edvinsson L. Cerebral autoregulation. Cerebrovascular and Brain Metabolism Reviews. 1990; 2:161-192

[24] Dickinson CJ. Why are strokes related to hypertension? Classic studies and hypotheses revisited. Journal of Hypertension. 2001;**19**:1515-1521

[25] Faraco G, Iadecola C. Hypertension: A harbinger of stroke and dementia. Hypertension. 2013;**62**:810-817

[26] Federico A, Di Donato I, Bianchi S, Di Palma C, Taglia I, Dotti MT. Hereditary cerebral small vessel diseases: A review. Journal of the Neurological Sciences. 2012;**322**(1-2): 25-30. DOI: 10.1016/j.jns.2012.07.041

[27] Pires PW, Dams Ramos CM, Matin N, Dorrance AM. The effects of hypertension on the cerebral circulation. American Journal of Physiology-Heart and Circulatory Physiology. 2013;**304**:1598-1614

[28] Hainsworth AH, Markus HS. Do in vivo experimental models reflect human cerebral small vessel disease? A systematic review. Journal of Cerebral Blood Flow and Metabolism. 2008; **28**:1877-1891

[29] Sierra C, Coca A, Schiffrin EL. Vascular mechanisms in the pathogenesis of stroke. Current Hypertension Reports. 2011;**13**(3):200-207. https://doi.org/10.1007/s11906-011-0195-x

[30] Sipahi I, Swaminathan A, Natesan V, Debanne SM, Simon DI, Fang JC. Effect of antihypertensive therapy on incident stroke in cohorts with prehypertensive blood pressure levels: A meta-analysis of randomized controlled trials. Stroke. 2012;**43**(2): 432-440. DOI: 10.1161/STROKEAHA. 111.636829

[31] Neal B, MacMahon S, Chapman N. Blood Pressure Lowering Treatment Trialists' Collaboration. Effects of ACE inhibitors, calcium antagonists, and other blood-pressure-lowering drugs: Results of prospectively designed overviews of randomised trials. The Lancet 2000;**356**(9246):1955-1964. DOI: 10.1016/s0140-6736(00) 03307-9.

[32] Meschia JF, Bushnell C, Boden-Albala B, Braun LT, Bravata DM, Chaturvedi S, et al. Guidelines for the primary prevention of stroke: A statement for healthcare professionals from the American Heart Association/ American Stroke Association. Stroke. 2014;**45**(12):3754-3832. DOI: 10.1161/ STR.0000000000000046

[33] Whelton PK, Carey RM, Aronow WS, Casey DE Jr, Collins KJ, Dennison Himmelfarb C, et al. 2017 ACC/AHA/AAPA/ABC/ACPM/AGS/ APhA/ASH/ASPC/NMA/PCNA guideline for the prevention, detection, evaluation, and management of high blood pressure in adults: Executive summary: A report of the American College of Cardiology/American Heart Association Task Force on clinical practice guidelines. Hypertension. 2018;**71**(6):1269-1324. DOI: 10.1161/ HYP.0000000000000066

[34] Williams B, Mancia G, Spiering W, Agabiti Rosei E, Azizi M, Burnier M, et al. Authors/Task Force Members: 2018 ESC/ESH guidelines for the management of arterial hypertension: The Task Force for the management of arterial hypertension of the European

Society of Cardiology and the European Society of Hypertension: Journal of Hypertension. 2018;**36**(10):1953-2041. DOI: 10.1097/HJH.0000000000001940.

[35] Gorelick PB, Aiyagari V. The management of hypertension for an acute stroke: What is the blood pressure goal? Current Cardiology Reports. 2013;**15**(6):366. DOI: 10.1007/s11886-013-0366-2

[36] Powers WJ, Rabinstein AA, Ackerson T, Adeoye OM, Bambakidis NC, Becker K, et al. Guidelines for the early management of patients with acute ischemic stroke: 2019 update to the 2018 guidelines for the early management of acute ischemic stroke: A guideline for healthcare professionals from the American Heart Association/American Stroke Association. Stroke. 2019;**50**(12): e344-e418. DOI: 10.1161/STR. 0000000000000211. Epub 2019 Oct 30. Erratum in: Stroke. 2019;50(12): e440-e441

[37] Sandset EC, Anderson CS, Bath PM, Christensen H, Fischer U, Gąsecki D, et al. European Stroke Organisation (ESO) guidelines on blood pressure management in acute ischaemic stroke and intracerebral haemorrhage. European Stroke Journal. 2021;**6**(2):II. DOI: 10.1177/23969873211026998

[38] Fischer U, Cooney MT, Bull LM, Silver LE, Chalmers J, Anderson CS, et al. Acute post-stroke blood pressure relative to premorbid levels in intracerebral haemorrhage versus major ischaemic stroke: A population-based study. Lancet Neurology. 2014;**13**(4): 374-384. DOI: 10.1016/S1474-4422 (14)70031-6

[39] Rodriguez-Luna D, Piñeiro S, Rubiera M, Ribo M, Coscojuela P, Pagola J, et al. Impact of blood pressure changes and course on hematoma growth in acute intracerebral hemorrhage. European Journal of

Neurology. 2013;**20**(9):1277-1283.
DOI: 10.1111/ene.12180

[40] Butcher KS, Jeerakathil T, Hill M,
Demchuk AM, Dowlatshahi D,
Coutts SB, et al. The intracerebral
hemorrhage acutely decreasing arterial
pressure trial. Stroke. 2013;**44**(3):620-
626. DOI: 10.1161/STROKEAHA.111.
000188

[41] Gould B, McCourt R, Asdaghi N,
Dowlatshahi D, Jeerakathil T, Kate M,
et al. Autoregulation of cerebral blood
flow is preserved in primary
intracerebral hemorrhage. Stroke.
2013;**44**(6):1726-1728. DOI: 10.1161/
STROKEAHA.113.001306

[42] Anderson CS, Heeley E, Huang Y,
Wang J, Stapf C, Delcourt C, et al. Rapid
blood-pressure lowering in patients with
acute intracerebral hemorrhage. The
New England Journal of Medicine. 2013;
368(25):2355-2365. DOI: 10.1056/
NEJMoa1214609

[43] Qureshi AI, Palesch YY, Barsan WG,
Hanley DF, Hsu CY, Martin RL, et al.
Intensive blood-pressure lowering in
patients with acute cerebral
hemorrhage. The New England Journal
of Medicine. 2016;**375**(11):1033-1043.
DOI: 10.1056/NEJMoa1603460

[44] Boulouis G, Morotti A,
Goldstein JN, Charidimou A. Intensive
blood pressure lowering in patients with
acute intracerebral haemorrhage:
clinical outcomes and haemorrhage
expansion. Systematic review and
meta-analysis of randomised trials.
Journal of Neurology, Neurosurgery,
and Psychiatry. 2017;**88**(4):339-345.
DOI: 10.1136/jnnp-2016-315346

[45] Lattanzi S, Cagnetti C,
Provinciali L, Silvestrini M. How should
we lower blood pressure after cerebral
hemorrhage? A systematic review and
meta-analysis. Cerebrovascular
Diseases. 2017;**43**(5-6):207-213.
DOI: 10.1159/000462986

[46] Gong S, Lin C, Zhang D, Kong X,
Chen J, Wang C, et al. Effects of
intensive blood pressure reduction on
acute intracerebral hemorrhage: A
systematic review and meta-analysis.
Scientific Reports. 2017;**7**(1):10694.
DOI: 10.1038/s41598-017-10892-z

[47] Shi L, Xu S, Zheng J, Xu J, Zhang J.
Blood pressure management for acute
intracerebral hemorrhage: A meta-
analysis. Scientific Reports. 2017;
7(1):14345. DOI: 10.1038/s41598-017-
13111-x

[48] Moullaali TJ, Wang X, Martin RH,
Shipes VB, Robinson TG, Chalmers J,
et al. Blood pressure control and clinical
outcomes in acute intracerebral
haemorrhage: A preplanned pooled
analysis of individual participant data.
Lancet Neurology. 2019;**18**(9):857-864.
DOI: 10.1016/S1474-4422(19)30196-6

[49] Qureshi AI, Huang W, Lobanova I,
Barsan WG, Hanley DF, Hsu CY, et al.
Outcomes of intensive systolic blood
pressure reduction in patients with
intracerebral hemorrhage and
excessively high initial systolic blood
pressure: Post hoc analysis of a
randomized clinical trial. JAMA
Neurology. 2020;**77**(11):1355-1365.
DOI: 10.1001/jamaneurol.2020.3075

[50] Hemphill JC 3rd, Greenberg SM,
Anderson CS, Becker K, Bendok BR,
Cushman M, et al. Guidelines for the
management of spontaneous
intracerebral hemorrhage: A guideline
for healthcare professionals from the
American Heart Association/American
Stroke Association. Stroke. 2015;**46**(7):
2032-2060. DOI: 10.1161/STR.0000000
000000069. Epub 2015 May 28

[51] Gorelick PB, Qureshi S,
Farooq MU. Management of blood
pressure in stroke. International Journal
of Cardiology: Hypertension.
2019;**3**:100021. DOI: 10.1016/j.ijchy.
2019.100021

[52] Feigin VL, Roth GA, Naghavi M, Parmar P, Krishnamurthi R, Chugh S, et al. Global burden of stroke and risk factors in 188 countries, during 1990-2013: A systematic analysis for the global burden of disease study 2013. Lancet Neurology. 2016;**15**:913-924. DOI: 10.1016/S1474-4422(16)30073-4

[53] Hackam DG, Spence JD. Combining multiple approaches for the secondary prevention of vascular events after stroke: A quantitative modeling study. Stroke. 2007;**38**:1881-1885. DOI: 10.1161/STROKEAHA.106.475525

[54] Kleindorfer DO, Towfighi A, Chaturvedi S, Cockroft KM, Gutierrez J, Lombardi-Hill D, et al. 2021 guideline for the prevention of stroke in patients with stroke and transient ischemic attack: A guideline from the American Heart Association/American Stroke Association. Stroke. 2021;**52**(7): e364-e467. DOI: 10.1161/STR.0000000000000375. Epub 2021 May 24. Erratum in: Stroke. 2021;52(7): e483-e484

[55] Prince M, Bryce R, Albanese E, Wimo A, Ribeiro W, Ferri CP. The global prevalence of dementia: A systematic review and metaanalysis. Alzheimer's & Dementia. 2013; **9**:63-75, e2. DOI: 10.1016/j.jalz.2012.11.007 [PubMed: 23305823]

[56] Toledo JB, Arnold SE, Raible K, Brettschneider J, Xie SX, Grossman M, et al. Contribution of cerebrovascular disease in autopsy confirmed neurodegenerative disease cases in the National Alzheimer's Coordinating Centre. Brain. 2013;**136**(Pt 9):2697-2706. DOI: 10.1093/brain/awt188

[57] Gorelick PB, Scuteri A, Black SE, Decarli C, Greenberg SM, Iadecola C, et al, On behalf of the American Heart Association Stroke Council, Council on Epidemiology and Prevention, Council on Cardiovascular Nursing, Council on Cardiovascular Radiology and Intervention, and Council on Cardiovascular Surgery and Anesthesia. Vascular contributions to cognitive impairment and dementia: A statement for healthcare professionals from the American Heart Association/American Stroke Association. Stroke. 2011; **42**:2672-2713

[58] Gąsecki D, Kwarciany M, Nyka W, Narkiewicz K. Hypertension, brain damage and cognitive decline. Current Hypertension Reports. 2013;**15**:547-558. DOI: 10.1007/s11906-013-0398-4

[59] Iadecola C, Gorelick PB. Converging pathogenic mechanisms in vascular and neurodegenerative dementia. Stroke. 2003;**34**:335-337

[60] Attems J, Jellinger KA. The overlap between vascular disease and Alzheimer's disease: Lessons from pathology. BMC Medicine. 2014;**12**:206. DOI: 10.1186/s12916-014-0206-2

[61] Schneider JA, Arvanitakis Z, Leurgans SE, Bennett DA. The neuropathology of probable Alzheimer disease and mild cognitive impairment. Annals of Neurology. 2009;**66**:200-208. DOI: 10.1002/ ana.21706

[62] Snowdon DA, Greiner LH, Mortimer JA, Riley KP, Greiner PA, Markesbery WR. Brain infarction and the clinical expression of Alzheimer disease: The Nun Study. Journal of the American Medical Association. 1997;**277**:813-817

[63] Chui HC, Zarow C, Mack WJ, Ellis WG, Zheng L, Jagust WJ, et al. Cognitive impact of subcortical vascular and Alzheimer's disease pathology. Annals of Neurology. 2006;**60**:677-687. DOI: 10.1002/ana.21009

[64] Chui HC, Ramirez-Gomez L. Clinical and imaging features of mixed Alzheimer and vascular pathologies.

Alzheimer's Research & Therapy. 2015;7:21. DOI: 10.1186/s13195-015-0104-7

[65] Norton S, Matthews FE, Barnes DE, Yaffe K, Brayne C. Potential for primary prevention of Alzheimer's disease: An analysis of population-based data [published correction appears in Lancet Neurology. 2014;13:1020]. Lancet Neurology. 2014;13:788-794. DOI: 10.1016/S1474-4422(14)70136-X

[66] Sierra C, Coca A. Brain damage. In: Mancia G, Grassi G, Redon J, editors. Manual of Hypertension of the European Society of Hypertension. 2nd ed. London: Informa Healthcare; 2014. pp. 177-189

[67] Manolio TA, Olson J, Longstreth WT. Hypertension and cognitive function: Pathophysiologic effects of hypertension on the brain. Current Hypertension Reports. 2003;5:255-261

[68] Rouch L, Cestac P, Hanon O, Cool C, Helmer C, Bouhanick B, et al. Antihypertensive drugs, prevention of cognitive decline and dementia: A systematic review of observational studies, randomized controlled trials and meta-analyses, with discussion of potential mechanisms. CNS Drugs. 2015;29(2):113-130. DOI: 10.1007/s40263-015-0230-6

[69] de Menezes ST, Giatti L, Brant LCC, Griep RH, Schmidt MI, Duncan BB, et al. Hypertension, prehypertension, and hypertension control: Association with decline in cognitive performance in the ELSA-Brasil cohort. Hypertension. 2021;77(2):672-681. DOI: 10.1161/HYPERTENSIONAHA.120.16080

[70] Forette F, Seux ML, Staessen JA, Thijs L, Birkenhäger WH, Babarskiene MR, et al. Prevention of dementia in randomised double-blind placebo-controlled systolic hypertension in Europe (Syst-Eur) trial. The Lancet. 1998;352(9137):1347-1351. DOI: 10.1016/s0140-6736(98)03086-4

[71] Tzourio C, Anderson C, Chapman N, Woodward M, Neal B, MacMahon S, et al. Effects of blood pressure lowering with perindopril and indapamide therapy on dementia and cognitive decline in patients with cerebrovascular disease. Archives of Internal Medicine. 2003;163(9):1069-1075. DOI: 10.1001/archinte.163.9.1069

[72] Barthold D, Joyce G, Wharton W, Kehoe P, Zissimopoulos J. The association of multiple anti-hypertensive medication classes with Alzheimer's disease incidence across sex, race, and ethnicity. PLoS One. 2018;13(11):e0206705. DOI: 10.1371/journal.pone.0206705

[73] Tu K, Anderson LN, Butt DA, Quan H, Hemmelgarn BR, Campbell NR, et al. Antihypertensive drug prescribing and persistence among new elderly users: Implications for persistence improvement interventions. The Canadian Journal of Cardiology. 2014;30(6):647-652. DOI: 10.1016/j.cjca.2014.03.017. Epub 2014 Mar 18

[74] Quitterer U, Abd Alla S. Improvements of symptoms of Alzheimer's disease by inhibition of the angiotensin system. Pharmacological Research. 2020;154:104230. DOI: 10.1016/j.phrs.2019.04.014

[75] Ungvari Z, Toth P, Tarantini S, Prodan CI, Sorond F, Merkely B, et al. Hypertension-induced cognitive impairment: From pathophysiology to public health. Nature Reviews Nephrology. 2021;14:1-16. DOI: 10.1038/s41581-021-00430-6

[76] Williamson JD, Pajewski NM, Auchus AP, Bryan RN, Chelune G, Cheung AK, et al. SPRINT MIND Investigators for the SPRINT Research Group. Effect of intensive vs standard blood pressure control on probable dementia: A randomized clinical trial.

JAMA. 2019 12;**321**(6):553-561. doi: 10.1001/jama.2018.21442.

[77] Waldstein SR, Giggey PP, Thayer JF, Zonderman AB. Nonlinear relations of blood pressure to cognitive function: The Baltimore longitudinal study of aging. Hypertension. 2005;**45**(3):374-379. DOI: 10.1161/01. HYP.0000156744.44218.74

[78] Lv YB, Zhu PF, Yin ZX, Kraus VB, Threapleton D, Chei CL, et al. A U-shaped association between blood pressure and cognitive impairment in Chinese elderly. Journal of the American Medical Directors Association. 2017 1;**18**(2):193.e7-193.e13. doi: 10.1016/j. jamda.2016.11.011.

[79] Hachinski V, Einhäupl K, Ganten D, Alladi S, Brayne C, Stephan BCM, et al. Preventing dementia by preventing stroke: The Berlin Manifesto. Alzheimer's & Dementia. 2019;**15**(7): 961-984. DOI: 10.1016/j.jalz.2019.06.001

[80] Friberg L, Rosenqvist M. Less dementia with oral anticoagulation in atrial fibrillation. European Heart Journal. 2018;**39**(6):453-460. DOI: 10.1093/eurheartj/ehx579

Section 2

Clinical and Diagnosis

Chapter 3

Atrial Fibrillation and Stroke

Francesca Spagnolo, Vincenza Pinto and Augusto Maria Rini

Abstract

Atrial fibrillation (AF) represents a major cause of morbidity and mortality in adults, especially for its strong association with thromboembolism and stroke. In this chapter, we aim to provide an overview on this cardiac arrhythmia, addressing several important questions. Particularly, we faced the possible mechanisms leading to an increased risk of embolism in AF, emphasizing how Virchow's triad for thrombogenesis is unable to fully explain this risk. Disentangling the risk of stroke caused by AF and by other associated vascular conditions is extremely challenging, and risk stratification of patients with AF into those at high and low risk of thromboembolism has become a crucial determinant of optimal antithrombotic prophylaxis. Moreover, we discuss the typical clinical and radiological characteristics of cardioembolic strokes, addressing acute, time-dependent reperfusional therapies in case of ischemic stroke. The role of anticoagulation in AF is also fully analyzed; the benefit of oral anticoagulation generally outweighs the risk of bleeding in AF patients, and a variety of scoring systems have been developed to improve clinical decision-making when initiating anticoagulation. With their predictable pharmacokinetic profiles, wide therapeutic windows, fewer drug–drug and drug-food interactions, and the non-vitamin K antagonist (VKA) oral anticoagulants (NOACs) have changed the landscape of thromboprophylaxis for AF patients, offering the opportunity to use effective anticoagulants without the need for intensive therapeutic drug monitoring.

Keywords: atrial fibrillation, stroke, ischemic, NAOS, prevention

1. Introduction

Thirty-three million people worldwide suffer from atrial fibrillation (AF), a common cardiac arrhythmia considered a major cause of morbidity and mortality in adults for its strong association with thromboembolism and stroke, which represents its most devastating complication [1].

AF is present in 3% of the general population above 20 years of age, and its prevalence increases substantially in people older than 65 years of age [2]. As expected, AF prevalence will increase as population get older [3].

Numerous cardiac pathologies, other than AF, have among their complications cardioembolic stroke. The cardiological substrate that is most frequently associated with embolism, especially in the elderly population, is represented by AF which is able to explain from 50% to 75% of all cerebral cardioembolic phenomena, in the West. AF may be caused by valvular, typically rheumatic, disease, but the vast majority of cases are of nonvalvular etiology. In this chapter, we will focus on nonvalvular AF.

The ischemic stroke rate among people with AF is about six times that of people without AF and varies greatly with coexisting cardiovascular disease. It is estimated that at least 15–20% of all ischemic strokes have a cardioembolic origin, carrying a mortality rate of 25% at 30 days and 50% at 1 year [4]. Strokes due to AF are often devastating: between 70% and 80% of patients die or have permanent disability [5, 6], but also largely preventable through anticoagulation, that guarantees a 64% reduction in stroke risk and a 25% reduction in mortality [7]. AF also increases the risk of cognitive impairment and dementia [8]. For these reasons, prevention of AF-related thromboembolic events must be a public health priority. However, since AF is often intermittent and asymptomatic, it can be easily undiagnosed [9, 10]. On the other hand, even dysrhythmic episodes of short duration seem to significantly increase the thromboembolic risk [11, 12] and deserve to be identified in order to be appropriately treated.

Therefore, risk stratification of patients with AF into those at high and low risk of thromboembolism has become a crucial determinant of optimal antithrombotic prophylaxis. This chapter will focus on discussing the deep association between this dysrhythmia and cerebrovascular accidents and identifying which patients with AF require long-term oral anticoagulation with either vitamin K antagonist (VKA; e.g. warfarin) or novel direct oral anticoagulants (DOAC).

2. Possible stroke mechanisms in AF

Only in 2% of patients with AF, no cardiac or extracardiac predisposing factor is detected, while 70% of AF cases are associated with organic heart diseases [13]. Risks factors associated with the development of AF are shown in **Table 1**.

The association between AF and ischemic stroke is strong and has been consistently confirmed in different cohorts [14–16]. After adjustment for risk factors, patients with AF face a three- to fivefold higher stroke risk than people without AF [14]. Therefore, a causal association between AF and stroke is biologically plausible, based on the assumption that in AF uncoordinated myocyte activity would lead to an impaired atrial contraction, stasis of blood and, as a result, to an increased thromboembolic risk. However, several other data do not support this straightforward relationship. For example, a clear biological gradient between the burden of AF and the risk of stroke is lacking: young and otherwise healthy patients with AF do not face a significantly increased stroke risk [17], while in older patients with vascular risk factors, a single brief episode of subclinical AF is associated with a twofold higher risk of stroke [9].

Moreover, the connection between AF and stroke also fails to respect the criterion of specificity: if AF causes thromboembolism, it should be specifically associated with embolic stroke. This is not the case, as for example 10% of patients with lacunar strokes have AF [18], and large-artery atherosclerosis is twice as common in patients with AF as those without [19].

Additionally, the criterion of temporality necessary to explain a causal relationship between AF and stroke is often not satisfied, and two recent studies found that approximately one-third of patients with both AF and stroke do not manifest any AF until after their stroke, despite undergoing continuous heart-rhythm monitoring before the cerebrovascular event [20, 21]. These data suggest that the mechanisms of stroke in AF have still to be fully elucidated and other factors are surely involved. Understanding the deep link between AF and stroke risk does

Major
• Hypertension
• Structural alterations of the heart (dilation and/or left ventricular hypertrophy, atriomegaly, valvulopathies, myo-pericarditis)
• Uncontrolled diabetes
• Heart failure
• Ischemic heart disease
• Old age

Minors
• Obesity
• History of atrial arrhythmias
• Lung diseases
• Thyroid diseases
• Smoke

Table 1.
Risk factors for atrial fibrillation.

not represent a pure academic exercise but has crucial therapeutic implications: if assuming that AF is the only cause of thromboembolism, maintaining normal rhythm should eliminate stroke risk. However, a recent meta-analysis of eight randomized clinical trials showed that a rhythm control strategy had no effect on stroke risk [22].

As in AF stroke risk cannot be entirely explained by the dysrhythmia itself, other factors are probably involved. Almost 150 years ago, Virchow hypothesized that development of thrombosis depends on three factors: abnormalities in blood flow, abnormalities in the blood vessel wall, and interaction with blood constituents [23]. Each of these elements may contribute to thromboembolism in AF [24, 25]. Dilated, poorly contracting atria, valvular heart disease (particularly mitral stenosis), and congestive heart failure represent abnormalities in blood flow and vessels, commonly associated with stroke and thromboembolism in patients with AF [24]. Independent clinical risk factors for stroke in nonvalvular AF also include a history of hypertension and diabetes, dilated left atrium, impaired left atrial function, and impaired left ventricular systolic function [26]. Aging and systemic vascular risk factors probably determine an abnormal atrial tissue substrate, or atrial cardiopathy, that can result in AF and/or thromboembolism [27]. Once AF develops, over time a structural remodeling of the atrium takes place, worsening atrial cardiopathy and further increasing the risk of thromboembolism, thereby propagating itself [28]. This mechanism can clarify why a brief period of AF is associated with stroke months later [9]. An *atrial substrate hypothesis* also explains the lack of specificity between AF and embolic stroke, as well as the fail of rhythm control strategies to eliminate thrombogenic potential. In this model, atrial cardiopathy alongside AF can cause thromboembolic stroke, explaining why one-third of strokes have no known cause [29], as well as why in many cryptogenic, cardioembolic, stroke only one-third of patients manifest AF even after 3 years of continuous heart-rhythm monitoring [30]. Supporting this hypothesis, a dilated left atrium and reduced left atrial and left atrial appendage (LAA) blood flow on echocardiography are independent risk factors for thromboembolism; the presence of spontaneous echo contrast or "smoke" on transesophageal echocardiography (TEE) is often observed in these patients. Spontaneous echo contrast has been related to hemodynamic and hemostatic abnormalities determining an increased risk of thromboembolism and stroke [31–36]. The presence of both left atrial spontaneous echo contrast and atrial enlargement in AF patients confer a very high risk of cerebral ischemic events (odds ratio 33.7) [34]. In this context, a greater emphasis on the atrial cardiopathy that led to AF may reinforce the importance of continuing proven anticoagulant treatments even after reoccurrence of normal rhythm.

Local epicardial fat and obesity-induced obstructive sleep apnea are increasingly recognized risk factors for atrial cardiopathy, contributing to local inflammation in the atrium, and raising intra-atrial pressures, respectively [37]. Intensive vascular risk factor management after AF ablation appears to improve the underlying atrial pathology [38].

Moreover, several observations indicate that AF is associated with a hyper-coagulable state [39]. Fibrin D-dimer levels are increased in patients with AF. In one study, fibrin D-dimer levels were highest in patients who were not receiving any antithrombotic therapy, intermediate in those onaspirin, and lowest in those treated with warfarin [40]. High-fibrin D-dimer levels have been associated with an increased rate of embolic events in patients with AF on oral anticoagulant (OAC) therapy [41, 42]. Endothelial damage and dysfunction in AF are also described [43–46]. Moreover, other data suggest that inflammation may contribute to the hypercoagulable state in AF [47]. As an example, high plasma levels of C-reactive protein (CRP) and interleukin-6 (IL-6) among patients with AF are independently related to indices of the prothrombotic state in AF (e.g. CRP to fibrinogen and IL-6 to tissue factor) [48]. In a larger series of 880 AF patients, CRP was positively correlated with stroke risk and prognosis, particularly mortality and vascular events [49]. Activation of the coagulation system has been identified by other authors in both paroxysmal [50, 51] and chronic AF [52, 53]. Cardioversion to sinus rhythm seems to result in normalization of hemostatic markers within 2–4 weeks [54]. Thereby, the mechanisms leading to an increased risk of stroke, thrombus, and embolism in AF are multiple, complex, and closely interact with each other. Many of these factors can be explained by Virchow's triad for thrombogenesis.

3. Factors increasing stroke risk in AF patients

Several conditions represent risk factors for both AF and stroke: age, gender (male sex), hypertension, diabetes mellitus, tobacco smoke, valvular hearth disease, heart failure, coronary heart disease, chronic kidney disease, inflammatory disorders, and sleep apnea confer higher risk of AF itself and stroke; disentangling the risk of stroke caused by AF and by these other associated conditions is challenging.

However, as we already said, AF remains independently associated with stroke even after adjusting for shared risk factors. Among conditions predisposing to thromboembolism in AF patients, particular attention has to be reserved to **cardioversion**. Cardioversion of AF leads to an increased risk of thromboembolism, particularly if patients are not anticoagulated before, during, and after cardioversion. In addition to dislodgement of preexisting thrombi, embolization may result from de novo thrombus formation induced by atrial contractile dysfunction after cardioversion, a transient condition known as atrial "stunning." This transient dysfunction has been described after spontaneous as well as drug or electrical restoration of normal rhythm, and its duration is at least partially related to the duration of AF, ranging from 24 hours to 1 week for AF duration lasting less than 2 weeks, and 2 to 6 weeks of AF, respectively. For longer periods of dysrhythmia, atrial stunning may last 1 month [55]. This long time of atrial dysfunction could explain why the great majority of embolic events in patients who remain in sinus rhythm occur within the first 10 days after cardioversion [56, 57].

Moreover, the presence of a poorly contracting, dilated left ventricle is likely to promote stasis of blood and lead to an increased risk of intracardiac thrombus formation and subsequent embolism. In fact, left ventricular dysfunction, i.e., heart failure, confers an additive risk of stroke to AF patients [58]. This risk is indirectly correlated with left ventricular ejection fraction (LVEF): every 5% point decrease in LVEF is associated with an 18% increase in the risk of stroke during a 42-month follow-up in patients with left ventricular dysfunction [58]. This risk was significantly reduced with the use of warfarin (relative risk 0.19) and oraspirin (relative risk 0.44).

As and probably more than in patients with AF, patients suffering from heart failure also demonstrate the presence of a prothrombotic or hypercoagulable state. As an example, both plasma fibrinogen and von Willebrand factor concentrations are often increased in heart failure, and platelet abnormalities are evident [59]. These blood dysfunctions may be additive to the hemodynamic and hemostatic abnormalities conferred by AF, further increasing the risk of thromboembolism [60].

Among valvular dysfunctions, mitral stenosis increases the risk of stroke in AF 17-fold [14]. On the other hand, the presence of mitral regurgitation seems to be protective against the development of intracardiac thrombi in chronic AF, presumably due to decreased stasis within the left atrium [24]. To support this hypothesis, the Stroke Prevention in Atrial Fibrillation (SPAF) study reported a decreased annual rate of clinical thromboembolism in patients with an enlarged left atrium and abnormal left ventricular wall motion if they also had mitral regurgitation (7.2% versus 15.4%) [61].

4. Characteristics of stroke in AF

AF is associated not just with stroke in general, but most strongly with strokes whose neuroimaging patterns resemble that of cardiac embolism [62]. Stroke associated with AF tends to be more extensive/larger than stroke related to carotid artery disease. This is probably due to embolization of larger thrombi with AF, which also explains "longer" transient ischemic attacks (TIAs) than emboli from carotid disease [63, 64].

Typical characteristics of cardioembolic strokes are the extension, bilaterality, the wedge-shaped appearance of the lesions, the presence of multiple vascular territories involved (particularly the lower division of the middle cerebral artery), and the rapid hemorrhagic transformation. Ischemic strokes with probable embolic pathophysiology cannot be clinically differentiated from ischemic strokes by other causes, although generally symptoms such as Wernicke's aphasia, homonymous lateral hemianopia without hemiparesis, and/or contralateral sensory deficit or an ideomotor apraxia are more suggestive of a cardioembolic origin [65]. Cardioembolic lesions generally present on MR images as multiple, narrow areas in DWI or CT scan involving several vascular districts and are generally bilateral. When a pattern with these characteristics is identified, an accurate evaluation of the heart becomes critical, taking into account all the possible sources of thromboembolism. At the same time when an isolated lesion in the territory of the anterior cerebral artery is documented on neuroimaging, a cardioembolic source should be considered, although the possibility of an atherosclerotic process involving the anterior cerebral artery itself (frequent in the Asian population, for example) is debated.

Patients with AF who suffer an ischemic stroke appear to have a worse outcome (the more the disability, the greater the mortality) than patients without AF [66, 67]. AF is also associated with silent cerebral infarctions and TIAs [68, 69] with an estimated rate of new silent cerebral infarcts of about 1.3% per year at up to 3 years of follow-up with a similar "silent" event rate for placebo and warfarin [68].

AF is asymptomatic in less than 40% of patients; unfortunately the absence of symptoms does not suggest a benign course [70], and stroke is the first manifestation of AF in at least 2–5% of patients [71]. In a hospital-based series, around 20% of stroke patients had previously unidentified or underrecognized AF [72]. Identifying AF and reducing stroke risk in patients with AF before stroke occurs is, therefore, an important goal.

5. Treatment and evalutation of acute ischemic stroke in AF patients

As we already said, the presence of AF in a stroke patient does not always mean that there is a causal relationship, and cerebral injuries, such as ischemic stroke affecting the autonomic nervous system can play an important role in the pathogenesis of AF itself [73]. In fact, several clinical observations support the hypothesis that stroke may trigger AF. For example, new-onset AF in stroke patients without left atrial enlargement may belong to this category [74]. However, even if stroke can trigger AF, this pathway cannot explain the well-documented association between AF and future stroke [14, 16], and one-third of patients with AF and stroke do not manifest AF until after their stroke [20]. For this reason, evaluation and treatment of stroke patients with AF is the same as the evaluation in other patients with acute stroke, including brain and neurovascular imaging, cardiac monitoring during the acute phase, and echocardiography. Patients with acute ischemic stroke should then be evaluated for possible reperfusion therapy even in the setting of AF, considering that international normalized ratio (INR) >1.7 or PT >15 s or evidence of intracranial hemorrhage (ICH) on neuroimaging are **absolute contraindications** to treatment with intravenous alteplase.

Current European guidelines [75] recommend that:

• for patients with acute ischemic stroke of <4.5 h duration, who use vitamin K antagonists and have INR lower than 1.7, intravenous thrombolysis with alteplase is indicated;

• for patients with acute ischemic stroke of <4.5 h duration, who use vitamin K antagonists and have INR >1.7, no intravenous thrombolysis is suggested;

• for patients with acute ischemic stroke of <4.5 h duration, alteplase is contraindicated if NOAC has been used during the last 48 h before stroke onset, according to the labels for these drugs [75].

Specific data on the risk/effectiveness balance of thrombolytic therapy in ischemic stroke patients suffering from AF are limited mainly to data coming from clinical trials [76, 77]. It seems to be no evidence of a treatment interaction between a history of AF and benefit from alteplase. The large size and worse prognosis of AF-associated acute ischemic stroke accentuates both the risks and the benefits of fibrinolysis [77]. In AF patients, mechanical thrombectomy is indicated as well, as in stroke without AF, when acute ischemic stroke is caused by an intracranial large-artery occlusion.

The detection of AF after stroke is important to delineate the mechanism of stroke itself and generally leads to a change in antithrombotic strategy. Long-term searching for AF allows to diagnose AF in 25% of patients with stroke or TIA [78];

most guidelines, therefore, recommend screening patients for the presence of AF, but the exact timing and duration of screening are undefined [79–82].

As a result of what we have said so far, if AF is a downstream marker of vascular risk factors that separately produce non-atrial stroke mechanisms, a comprehensive approach to the patient, with full consideration of other causes of stroke, is desirable. Moreover emphasizing intensive management of all risk factor is a crucial point to stroke secondary prevention.

6. Role of anticoagulation in AF

Thromboprophylaxis is critical for stroke prevention in AF patients. Despite overwhelming evidence that oral anticoagulation is superior to aspirin for primary stroke prevention in patients with AF, aspirin remains overused; notwithstanding, it is only minimally effective and confers a bleeding risk that is similar to that of well-controlled warfarin [7, 83–85]. This evidence is underlined in the recent National Institute for Health and Care Excellence (NICE) [86] and European Society of Cardiology guidelines [87]. Ischemic stroke can occur with either paroxysmal (intermittent) or chronic (permanent) AF. Long-term anticoagulation is recommended to reduce the risk of thromboembolism for most patients with AF, but its use is associated with and increased risk of bleeding. However, the benefit generally outweighs the risk, and randomized trials have shown that therapeutic oral anticoagulant (OAC) reduces the risk of ischemic stroke and other embolic events by approximately two-thirds compared with placebo, irrespective of baseline risk [84, 88–95]. Moreover anticoagulated AF patients who experience ischemic stroke typically have smaller infarcts and lower mortality rates compared with not anticoagulated AF patients [96]. A variety of scoring systems have been developed to evaluate the risks of thrombosis and bleeding, thus aiding clinical decision-making when initiating anticoagulation [97, 98].

With their predictable pharmacokinetic profiles, wide therapeutic windows, and fewer drug–drug and drug-food interactions, the non-VKA oral anticoagulants (NOACs) have changed the landscape of thromboprophylaxis for ischemic stroke, offering physicians and patients the opportunity to use effective anticoagulants without the need for intensive therapeutic drug monitoring. The NOACs have been shown to be noninferior to warfarin for stroke prevention in patients with AF, although each has various properties that may favor use in particular patients, allowing physicians to fit the drug to patient's profile [99–102]. As the therapeutic armamentarium for the management of ischemic stroke risk in AF has expanded, clinical decision-making in terms of the choice of anticoagulant has become more complex.

Warfarin. Slow onset, drug–drug and drug-food interactions [103], genetic polymorphisms in CYP2C9 [104], and the vitamin K epoxide reductase complex subunit [105], all affect the anticoagulant effect of warfarin, making it monitoring of the international normalized ratio (INR) sometimes very difficult. Even when an optimal control of anticoagulation is achieved, adverse hemorrhagic events can still occur in patients treated with VKAs. However, warfarin is the most studied antithrombotic therapy for the prevention of recurrent stroke in patients with AF. A meta-analysis including six randomized trials comparing warfarin with placebo or no treatment in a total of 2900 participants with AF showed that the overall rate of stroke was 2.2%/patient year in the warfarin group and 6.0%/patient year in the control group (relative risk reduction 0.64; 95% CI 0.49–0.74) [7]. With warfarin therapy, all-cause mortality was reduced by 1.6%/year (relative risk reduction 0.26; 95% CI 0.03–0.43). Compared with aspirin, treatment with adjusted-dose warfarin

(INR between 2 and 3) reduced stroke risk in AF patients from 10% to 4% per year in a pooled analysis of several randomized trials [84].

Direct oral anticoagulants (DOACs), also referred to as **non-vitamin K oral anticoagulants (NOACs)**, have been less extensively studied but appear to be equally efficacious than warfarin in stroke prevention. These drugs were developed to provide efficacious anticoagulation with rapid onset, a favorable side effect profile and predictable pharmacokinetic properties, obviating the need for therapeutic drug monitoring [106–108]. Two classes of NOACs have been developed: the direct thrombin inhibitors (Dabigatran [100]) and the direct factor Xa inhibitors (Rivaroxaban [101], Apixaban [99], and Edoxaban [102]; **Table 2**). All four agents have been found to be individually noninferior to warfarin for the prevention of stroke and systemic embolism in large, international randomized trials [99–102]. However, to date, there is no evidence to suggest that any of the NOACs are superior to the others for the prevention of stroke in AF.

Apixaban—Apixaban was compared with adjusted-dose warfarin in the ARISTOTLE trial, demonstrating to be even superior to warfarin in preventing stroke or systemic embolism (1.3% versus 1.6%) [109]. Apixaban also caused less major bleeding compared with warfarin (2.1% versus 3.1%) and resulted in lower overall mortality (3.5% versus 3.9%) [109]. Moreover, preliminary secondary analysis of data from the AUGUSTUS trial that enrolled patients suggested a superiority of apixaban to vitamin K antagonists with regard to intracranial bleeding and stroke/TIA/thromboembolism in AF patients with a recent acute coronary syndrome and a prior stroke/TIA/thromboembolism [110].

Dabigatran—Dabigatran was compared with adjusted-dose warfarin in a trial involving over 18,000 AF patients [100]. Dabigatran compared favorably to warfarin, including in the subset of participants with prior stroke.

Edoxaban—A trial comparing edoxaban 15 mg daily with placebo in patients with AF ≥80 years old with low body weight found a similar relative reduction in risk of stroke or systemic embolism than warfarin (2.3% versus 6.7%/year; hazard

	Warfarin	Dabigatran	Rivaroxaban	Apixaban	Edoxaban
Target:	Synthesis of factors vitamin coagulation K-employees (II, VII, IX, X)	Trombina	Factor Xa	Factor Xa	Factor Xa
Bioavailability:	100%	6.5% (absolute)	80%	50% (absolute)	60% (absolute)
Food effect:	None	Delayed, not reduced	Increased (20 mg)	None	None
Protein binding:	99%	35%	>90%	87%	40–59%
Prodrug:	No	Yes	No	No	No
C_{max} (h):	2–4	1–3	2–4	3–4	2
Half-life time (h):	40	12–17	5–9 (healthy)	8–15	8–11
Renal elimination:	0%	80%	65%	27%	35%
Administration:	Single dose daily	Double dose daily	Single dose daily	Double dose daily	Single dose daily

Table 2.
Main pharmacokinetic characteristics of warfarin and the new oral anticoagulants.

ratio (HR) 0.34, 95% CI 0.19–0.61) [111]. Edoxaban was compared with warfarin in the ENGAGE TIMI 48 trial of over 21,000 patients [102]. Edoxaban was found to be noninferior with regard to the primary efficacy end point and caused less bleeding.

Rivaroxaban—Rivaroxaban was found to be non-inferior to warfarin in the ROCKET AF trial in preventing stroke or noncentral nervous systemic embolism [101].

7. Risk stratification

Despite the advantages, OAC therapy is associated with an increased risk of bleeding. Then, benefit and risk ration must be taken into account to identify patients with AF who are likely to benefit from OAC. For each patient, the estimated absolute risk reduction for thromboembolic events is weighed against the estimated increase in absolute risk of intracranial hemorrhage and other major bleeding complications, along with patient preferences.

If AF develops, females are more symptomatic and at higher risk of thrombo-embolism than males. This is particularly true for age older than 65 years. In fact, female AF patients have an increased risk of stroke, aggravated by the lower oral anticoagulant prescription rate correlated with the concomitant higher bleeding risk profile. Catheter ablation is underutilized in female patients and, conversely, they are more commonly affected by the side effects of antiarrhythmic drugs [112].

To estimate thromboembolic risk in patients with AF, a variety of risk scores and biomarkers have been studied [113]. Unfortunately, imaging findings have not been shown to improve risk stratification in patients with AF [114].

The CHA_2DS_2-VASc score (**Table 3**) has been compared with other potential alternatives, resulting as the most accurate in identifying patients at lowest risk for thromboembolism.

The decision whether to prescribe OAC in AF should be based upon risk assessment, according to the following risk stratification:

- For a CHA2DS2-VASc score ≥ 2 in males or ≥ 3 in females, chronic OAC is recommended; [115–118].

- For a CHA2DS2-VASc score of 1 in males and 2 in females:

    1. Patients between 65 to 74 years old, with CHA2DS2-VASc score of 1 in males and 2 in females, OAC is recommended [119].

    2. For patients with other risk factors, the decision to anticoagulated is based upon the specific nonsex risk factor and the burden of AF. For patients with very low burden of AF (e.g., AF that is well documented as limited to an isolated episode that may have been due to a reversible cause), it may be reasonable to institute close surveillance for recurrent AF.

- For patients with a CHA2DS2-VASc score of 0 in males and 1 in females, no anticoagulant therapy should be started, as thromboembolic risk is low [112].

According to the CHA_2DS_2-VASc score, anticoagulation is generally recommended for individuals with all but the lowest level of risk. The annual risk of ischemic stroke in untreated patients is estimated to be 0.2%, 0.6%, and 2.2% for those with CHA_2DS_2-VASc scores of 0, 1, and 2, respectively [115].

Unfortunately, the CHA_2DS_2-VASc score has several limitations: the risk associated with older age is not continuous, but lumped into categories, so that, for

Clinical criteria	
Sex	
Female	1 point
Male	0 point
Age	
<64 years old	0 point
65–74 years old	1 point
>75 years old	2 points
Comorbidities	
Heart failure	1 point
Hypertension	1 point
Diabetes mellitus	1 point
History of stroke, TIA, or thromboembolism	2 points
Vascular disease (history of MI, PAD, or aortic atherosclerosis)	1 point
Unadjusted stroke rate:	
0 point: 0.2% per year	
1 point: 0.6% per year	
2 points: 2.2% per year	
3 points: 3.2% per year	
4 points: 4.8% per year	
5 points: 7.2% per year	
6 points: 9.7% per year	
7 points: 11.2% per year	
8 points: 10.8% per year	
9 points 12.2% per year	

Table 3.
CHA2DS2-VASc risk stratification score.

example, ages 65 years and 74 years each confer one point, despite the much higher actual risk associated with the older age. A history of prior stroke, transient ischemic attack, or thromboembolic event is assigned two points, but the risk associated with this risk factor is more than five times the risk associated with risk factors assigned one point. Risk factors assigned equal point values are associated with substantially different risks, and, again, ages between 65 and 74 years are associated with substantially greater stroke risk than other risk factors assigned one point.

A recent systematic review found that nonpermanent forms of AF may have a 25% lower risk of stroke compared with permanent forms of AF [120]. Short episodes of AF may occur in 30–60% of monitored patients [121]; however, their relevance is particularly questioned, especially regarding the duration of AF required to increase the risk of stroke independently from the general cardiovascular risk profile [122]. A post hoc analysis of the ASSERT trial (Asymptomatic Atrial Fibrillation and Stroke Evaluation in Pacemaker Patients and the AF Reduction Atrial Pacing trial) suggest that only episodes lasting longer than 24 h are relevant and carry a threefold risk of future thromboembolism over the next 2.5 years [123]. However, the AF burden (duration and frequency of episodes) is likely to vary over time, while a large proportion of patients with short episodes of AF will go on to experience longer episodes, it is also true that the reverse occurs in a percentage of patients experiencing long episodes of AF [124]. Moreover, the extent to which thromboembolic risk may continue during periods of sinus rhythm is uncertain. As discussed earlier, the risk of thromboembolism is not reduced by clinical maintenance of sinus rhythm.

Unfortunately, so far none of the risk stratification schemes and guidelines have incorporated the type of AF or have adopted a different stance toward recommending anticoagulation in patients with paroxysmal AF.

Some clinical features or conditions may impact the risk of thromboembolism but are not included in risk models; these include the presence of conditions such as chronic kidney disease and elevated troponin level. Prediabetes has also been implicated as a possible risk factor for stroke in patients with AF [125].

AF is often diagnosed in the context of systemic conditions like pneumonia and thyroid disease or after cardiothoracic surgery [126]. In these patients, anticoagulation is not typically advised for the transitorily of the condition. However, recent data suggest that these patients are at high risk of recurrent AF and stroke [126–128]. Whether patients with secondary AF will benefit from early anticoagulation or should undergo repeated screening for AF is currently unknown [129].

8. Risk of bleeding

For all potential candidates for OAC, bleeding risk and related possible contraindications to OAC should be carefully considered, especially for modifiable bleeding risk factors and to identify patients that rather than from OAC could benefit from left atrial appendage occlusion [112, 114, 130].

The major safety concern is risk of major bleeding, which includes events that require hospitalization, transfusion, or surgery, or that involve particularly sensitive anatomic locations, as intracranial bleeding. Among patients with AF, the three most important predictors of major bleeding (including ICH) are over-anticoagulation with warfarin (defined as an international normalized ratio greater than 3.0), prior stroke, and older patient age [116, 131].

ICH is the most serious bleeding complication, since the likelihood of mortality or subsequent major disability is substantially higher than with bleeding at other sites, and similar to that for ischemic stroke [132].

The HAS-BLED risk score (**Table 4**), based upon bleeding risk with warfarin, is the best predictor of bleeding risk [114] and can be used to identify patients at high risk of hemorrhage [98].

The annual risk of intracranial bleeding with warfarin is around 0.3%. Compared to warfarin, each of the NOACs dramatically reduces the incidence of intracranial hemorrhage [133], with subtle differences between NOACs regarding other types of major hemorrhage. Low-dose dabigatran (RR 0.80, 95% CI 0.69–0.93; $P = 0.003$), apixaban (RR 0.69, 95% CI 0.60–0.80; $P < 0.001$), and edoxaban at high (RR 0.80, 95% CI 0.70–0.91; $P < 0.001$) and low dose (RR 0.47, 95% CI 0.41–0.55; $P < 0.001$) have demonstrated a significant reduced rate of major hemorrhage compared to warfarin, while high-dose dabigatran and rivaroxaban seem equivalent to warfarin in terms of the incidence of major hemorrhage. In summary, in patients at high risk of gastrointestinal hemorrhage, it is reasonable to avoid high-dose dabigatran and high-dose edoxaban and rivaroxaban [133]; low-dose edoxaban may be preferred. In patients with high HAS-BLED scores who have suffered major hemorrhage, low-dose dabigatran, apixaban, and edoxaban are all appropriate choices of anticoagulant, but the risk of hemorrhage should be balanced carefully against the risk of stroke and patients' personal preferences.

	Clinical characteristics	Points
H	Hypertension	1
A	Abnormal renal or liver function (1 point each)	1–2
S	Stroke	1
B	Bleeding tendency or predisposition	1
L	Labile INR (for patients taking warfarin)	1
E	Elderly (age greater than 65 years)	1
D	Drugs (concomitant aspirin or NSAIDs) or excess alcohol use (1 point each)	1–2
		Maximum 9

HAS-BLED score	
Total points	Bleeds per 100 patient-years
0	1.13
1	1.02
2	1.88
3	3.74
4	8.70
>5	Insufficient data

Table 4.
HAS-BLED bleeding risk score.

9. Alternatives to anticoagulation

9.1 Left atrial appendage occlusion

It represents the primary alternative to long-term anticoagulation for patients with AF.

9.2 Pharmacologic agents

As we already said, no other antithrombotic regimen is as effective as chronic oral anticoagulation in AF patients. However, despite being less effective, in specific clinical setting, other antithrombotic regimens have to be considered in order to lower thromboembolic risk. Given the availability of the new class of anticoagulant agents, as alternatives to vitamin K antagonists, this situation should be extremely uncommon.

9.2.1 Aspirin plus clopidogrel

In patients with AF, dual antiplatelet therapy (with aspirin plus clopidogrel) reduces the risk of thromboembolism compared with aspirin monotherapy but offers less protection against thromboembolism than OAC. So, dual antiplatelet therapy is preferred to aspirin alone in the occasional high-risk patient with AF who cannot be treated with any OAC for a reason other than risk of bleeding. Of note, dual antiplatelet therapy and OAC have similar bleeding risks [134, 135].

9.2.2 Aspirin monotherapy

Aspirin (or other antiplatelet agent) is not an effective therapy for preventing thromboembolic events in patients with AF. The role of aspirin alone in lowering the risk of stroke and systemic embolism in patients with AF is not confirmed in all meta-analyses of clinical trials [7, 113, 136]. In contrast, clinical trials have clearly demonstrated that OAC (with VKA or DOAC) lowers the risk of thromboembolism compared with aspirin [7, 84, 89, 92, 137].

9.2.3 Aspirin plus low-dose warfarin

Low-dose warfarin (1.25 mg/day or target INR between 1.2 and 1.5) in combination with aspirin (300 to 325 mg/day) should not be used to reduce stroke risk in patients with nonvalvular AF [95, 138, 139].

10. Stroke while on anticoagulation

Subtherapeutic anticoagulation and low compliance are the most common causes of treatment failure for patients taking warfarin and DOAC, respectively. Due to NOACs short half-lives, adherence to medication is of great importance and missed doses can lead to suboptimal anticoagulant effect and increased risk of stroke. Considerations about patient's compliance are essential when prescribing a twice-daily (dabigatran and apixaban) or once-daily regimen (rivaroxaban and edoxaban). However, in all AF patients experiencing a new ischemic cerebrovascular event while on OAC, a non-cardioembolic stroke mechanism (e.g., lacunar, large-artery stenosis, and malignancy) should be suspected. In case of a subtherapeutic anticoagulation (INR < 2) while on warfarin, continuing warfarin with renewed efforts to keep the INR in the therapeutic range (INR 2–3) or consideration of a change to a DOAC is recommended. When ischemic stroke occurs with a therapeutic INR (2–3), it is reasonable to perform a transesophageal echocardiogram (TEE) to assess for left atrial appendage (LAA) thrombus, though in these cases the ischemic stroke is often "lacunar," related to cerebral small artery disease, rather than cardioembolic. Increasing the target INR to 2.5–3.5 and switching from warfarin to a DOAC are both possible therapeutic strategies. Addition of antiplatelet therapy is generally not recommended, as it is known to increase major hemorrhage, particularly intracranial hemorrhage, and the benefit is not well defined. While data are limited, ischemic stroke during therapy with a DOAC for AF has been associated with several factors, including treatment at doses lower than recommended. Continuing anticoagulation therapy is generally indicated. If a thrombus is present despite appropriate dosing and compliance, it is reasonable to change to another DOAC, but optimal treatment is uncertain and no consensus exists. A retrospective study suggested that for patients with left ventricular thrombus, warfarin may be superior to DOAC for reducing the risk of stroke or systemic embolism. Unfortunately, analogous data for AF patients with left atrial appendage thrombi are lacking. As we already said, limited available data suggest that there is no benefit from adding aspirin to therapeutic OAC in patients with AF.

10.1 Timing after acute ischemic stroke

For medically stable patients with a small- or moderate-sized infarct with no intracranial bleeding, warfarin can be initiated soon (after 24 h) after admission with minimal risk of transformation to hemorrhagic stroke. As DOAC have a more rapid anticoagulant effect than warfarin, usually in these patients they are initiated after 48 h since ischemic stroke. Withholding anticoagulation for 2 weeks is generally recommended for those with large ischemic strokes [140], symptomatic hemorrhagic transformation, or poorly controlled hypertension. Patients who are not treated with warfarin earlier may benefit from aspirin until therapeutic anticoagulation is achieved [141].

10.2 Secondary prevention in patients with AF

A recent meta-analysis of the RE-LY, ROCKET-AF, and ARISTOTLE trials demonstrated that dabigatran, rivaroxaban, and apixaban were all noninferior to warfarin in the secondary prevention of stroke in patients with AF [142].

Apixaban seems to confer the lowest risk of stroke or systemic embolism in patients who had already suffered a previous ischemic cerebrovascular event (RR 0.77, 95% CI 0.57–1.03); however, this finding was not statistically significant [99]. In the four major clinical trials of NOACs compared with warfarin, patients were stratified by stroke risk using the CHADS2 score. Both high-dose dabigatran (150 mg b.d.) (RR 0.73, 95% CI 0.58–0.91; $P = 0.005$) and apixaban (HR 0.79, 95% CI 0.66–0.95; $P = 0.01$ for superiority) demonstrated superiority to warfarin in the prevention of stroke and systemic embolism [99]. However, so far, evidences are not strong enough to suggest the NOACs are superior to warfarin in the secondary prevention of stroke in patients with AF.

11. AF and older age

The consequences of AF are particularly pronounced in older individuals. In patients with documented frequent falls, the risks/benefits ratio of OAC should be carefully evaluated, and working to reduce the risk of falls is recommended. The risk of falls leading to subdural hematomas is increased in older adult patients taking oral anticoagulants independent of the agent chosen. A Taiwanese database study compared 15,756 older (≥90 years of age) adults with AF (11,064 receiving no antithrombotic therapy, 4075 receiving antiplatelet therapy, and 617 on warfarin) with 14,658 older adult patients without AF and without antithrombotic therapy [143]. In this study, patients with AF had a greater risk of ischemic stroke (5.75 versus 3.00%/year; hazard ratio [HR] 1.93, 95% CI 1.74–2.14) and a similar risk of intracranial hemorrhage (ICH; 0.97 versus 0.54%/year; HR 0.85, 95% CI 0.66–1.09) compared with those without AF. Among patients with AF, warfarin use was associated with a lower stroke risk (3.83% versus 5.75%/year; HR 0.69, 95% CI 0.49–0.96) compared with no antithrombotic therapy. There was a nominal but nonsignificant increase in risk of ICH (HR 1.26, 95% CI 0.70–2.25). In a second, later cohort of patients ≥90 years of age with AF, 768 patients treated with warfarin were compared with 978 patients treated with a direct oral anticoagulant (DOAC) [143]. DOACs were associated with a lower risk of ICH compared with warfarin (0.42% versus 1.63%/year; HR 0.32, 95% CI 0.10–0.97) and similar rate of ischemic stroke (4.07% versus 4.59%/year; HR 1.16; 95% CI 0.61–2.22).

12. Final remarks

To date, we know that atrial fibrillation is the result of a complex interplay between genetic predisposition, ectopic electrical activity, and abnormal tissue pathology; AF is able to propagate itself feeding back to remodel and worsen tissue substrate. However, despite our understanding, the prevailing model of AF and thromboembolism is likely incomplete, and new strategies for identifying and treating patients at risk of thromboembolism are needed. More work is especially required to determine whether additional markers, such as cardiac magnetic resonance imaging of tissue fibrosis and computed tomographic assessment of left atrial appendage morphology, may better identify the risk of atrial thromboembolism. The advent of NOACs have revolutionized the management of AF patients offering predictable, easy-to-use drugs that show similar efficacy than warfarin for stroke prevention, but lower rates of intracranial hemorrhage. However, despite the availability of these new drugs, selecting and adhering to anticoagulant therapy remains challenging for physicians and patients with AF. Further studies are needed to explore NOACs use, empowering physicians to manage stroke risk especially in high-risk patients, providing a subject-centered, tailored approach to the management of thromboembolic risk in AF patients.

Abbreviations

NOAC	novel oral anticoagulants
MR	Magnetic Resonance
MI	Myocardial Infarction
PAD	peripheral artery disease

Author details

Francesca Spagnolo*, Vincenza Pinto and Augusto Maria Rini
Department of Neurology, Antonio Perrino's Hospital, Brindisi, Italy

*Address all correspondence to: francesca.spagnolo81@gmail.com

IntechOpen

References

[1] Chugh SS, Havmoeller R, Narayanan K, Singh D, Rienstra M, Benjamin EJ, et al. Worldwide epidemiology of atrial fibrillation: A global burden of disease 2010 study. Circulation. 2014;**129**:837-847 [PubMed: 24345399]

[2] Rahman F, Kwan GF, Benjamin EJ. Global epidemiology of atrial fibrillation. Nature Reviews. Cardiology. 2014;**11**:639-654. DOI: 10.1038/nrcardio.2014.118

[3] Naccarelli GV, Varker H, Lin J, Schulman KL. Increasing prevalence of atrial fibrillation and flutter in the United States. The American Journal of Cardiology. 2009;**104**:1534-1539

[4] Zhang H, Li Z, Dai Y, et al. Ischemic stroke etiological classification system: The agreement analysis of CISS, SPARKLE and TOAST. Stroke and Vascular Neurology. 2019;**4**(3):123-128

[5] Gladstone DJ, Bui E, Fang J, et al. Potentially preventable strokes in high-risk patients with atrial fibrillation who are not adequately anticoagulated. Stroke. 2009;**40**:235-240

[6] Saposnik G, Gladstone D, Raptis R, Zhou L, Hart RG. Investigators of the Registry of the Canadian Stroke Network (RCSN) and the Stroke Outcomes Research Canada (SORCan) Working Group. Atrial fibrillation in ischemic stroke: Predicting response to thrombolysis and clinical outcomes. Stroke. 2013;**44**:99-104

[7] Hart RG, Pearce LA, Aguilar MI. Meta-analysis: Antithrombotic therapy to prevent stroke in patients who have nonvalvular atrial fibrillation. Annals of Internal Medicine. 2007;**146**:857-867

[8] Singh-Manoux A, Fayosse A, Sabia S, Canonico M, Bobak M, Elbaz A, et al. Atrial fibrillation as a risk factor for cognitive decline and dementia. European Heart Journal. 2017;**38**(34): 2612-2618. DOI: 10.1093/eurheartj/ehx208

[9] Healey JS, Connolly SJ, Gold MR, et al. Subclinical atrial fibrillation and the risk of stroke. The New England Journal of Medicine. 2012;**366**:120-129

[10] Camm AJ, Corbucci G, Padeletti L. Usefulness of continuous electrocardiographic monitoring for atrial fibrillation. The American Journal of Cardiology. 2012;**110**:270-276

[11] Hohnloser SH, Pajitnev D, Pogue J, et al. Incidence of stroke in paroxysmal versus sustained atrial fibrillation in patients taking oral anticoagulation or combined antiplatelet therapy: An AC-TIVE W substudy. Journal of the American College of Cardiology. 2007;**50**:2156-2161

[12] Gaita F, Corsinovi L, Anselmino M, et al. Prevalence of silent cerebral ischemia in paroxysmal and persistent atrial fibrillation and correlation with cognitive function. Journal of the American College of Cardiology. 2013;**62**:1990-1997

[13] Schoonderwoerd B, Smith MD, Pen L, et al. New risks factors for atrial fibrillation: Cause of "not-so-lone atrial fibrillation". Europace. 2008;**10**:668-673

[14] Wolf PA, Dawber TR, Thomas HE Jr, Kannel WB. Epidemiologic assessment of chronic atrial fibrillation and risk of stroke: The Framingham study. Neurology. 1978;**28**:973

[15] Hill AB. The environment and disease: Association or causation? Proceedings of the Royal Society of Medicine. 1965;**58**:295-300 [PubMed: 14283879]

[16] Manolio TA, Kronmal RA, Burke GL, O'Leary DH, Price TR.

Short-term predictors of incident stroke in older adults. The Cardiovascular Health Study. Stroke. 1996;27:1479-1486 [PubMed: 8784116]

[17] Chao TF, Liu CJ, Chen SJ, Wang KL, Lin YJ, Chang SL, et al. Atrial fibrillation and the risk of ischemic stroke: Does it still matter in patients with a CHA2DS2-VASc score of 0 or 1? Stroke. 2012;43:2551-2555 [PubMed: 22871677]

[18] Lodder J, Bamford JM, Sandercock PA, Jones LN, Warlow CP. Are hypertension or cardiac embolism likely causes of lacunar infarction? Stroke. 1990;21:375-381 [PubMed: 2309260]

[19] Chesebro JH, Fuster V, Halperin JL. Atrial fibrillation--risk marker for stroke. The New England Journal of Medicine. 1990;323:1556-1558 [PubMed: 2233936]

[20] Brambatti M, Connolly SJ, Gold MR, Morillo CA, Capucci A, Muto C, et al. Temporal relationship between subclinical atrial fibrillation and embolic events. Circulation. 2014;129:2094-2099 [PubMed: 24633881]

[21] Martin DT, Bersohn MM, Waldo AL, Wathen MS, Choucair WK, Lip GY, et al. Randomized trial of atrial arrhythmia monitoring to guide anticoagulation in patients with implanted defibrillator and cardiac resynchronization devices. European Heart Journal. 2015;36:1660-1668 [PubMed: 25908774]

[22] Al-Khatib SM, Allen LaPointe NM, Chatterjee R, Crowley MJ, Dupre ME, Kong DF, et al. Rate- and rhythm-control therapies in patients with atrial fibrillation: A systematic review. Annals of Internal Medicine. 2014;160:760-773 [PubMed: 24887617]

[23] Virchow R. Gesammelte abhandlungen zur wissenschaftlichen medizin. Frankfurt: Medinger Sohn & Co; 1856. p. 219

[24] Lip GY, Lowe GD. ABC of atrial fibrillation. Antithrombotic treatment for atrial fibrillation. British Medical Journal. 1996;312:45

[25] Lip GY, Lowe GD, Rumley A, Dunn FG. Increased markers of thrombogenesis in chronic atrial fibrillation: Effects of warfarin treatment. British Heart Journal. 1995;73:527

[26] Predictors of thromboembolism in atrial fibrillation: II. Echocardiographic features of patients at risk. The stroke prevention in Atrial fibrillation Investigators. Annals of Internal Medicine. 1992;116:6

[27] Kamel H, Okin PM, Elkind MSV, Iadecola C. Atrial fibrillation and mechanisms of stroke: Time for a new model. Stroke. 2016;47(3):895-900

[28] Heijman J, Voigt N, Nattel S, Dobrev D. Cellular and molecular electrophysiology of atrial fibrillation initiation, maintenance, and progression. Circulation Research. 2014;114: 1483-1499 [PubMed: 24763466]

[29] Marnane M, Duggan CA, Sheehan OC, Merwick A, Hannon N, Curtin D, et al. Stroke subtype classification to mechanism-specific and undetermined categories by TOAST, A-S-C-O, and causative classification system. Stroke. 2010;41:1579-1586 [PubMed: 20595675]

[30] Sanna T, Diener HC, Passman RS, Di Lazzaro V, Bernstein RA, Morillo CA, et al. Cryptogenic stroke and underlying atrial fibrillation. The New England Journal of Medicine. 2014;370:2478-2486 [PubMed: 24963567]

[31] Black IW, Hopkins AP, Lee LC, Walsh WF. Left atrial spontaneous echo contrast: A clinical and echocardiographic analysis. Journal of

the American College of Cardiology. 1991;**18**:398

[32] Black IW, Chesterman CN, Hopkins AP, et al. Hematologic correlates of left atrial spontaneous echo contrast and thromboembolism in nonvalvular atrial fibrillation. Journal of the American College of Cardiology. 1993;**21**:451

[33] Daniel WG, Nellessen U, Schröder E, et al. Left atrial spontaneous echo contrast in mitral valve disease: An indicator for an increased thromboembolic risk. Journal of the American College of Cardiology. 1988;**11**:1204

[34] Jones EF, Calafiore P, McNeil JJ, et al. Atrial fibrillation with left atrial spontaneous contrast detected by transesophageal echocardiography is a potent risk factor for stroke. The American Journal of Cardiology. 1996;**78**:425

[35] Heppell RM, Berkin KE, McLenachan JM, Davies JA. Haemostatic and haemodynamic abnormalities associated with left atrial thrombosis in non-rheumatic atrial fibrillation. Heart. 1997;**77**:407

[36] Bernhardt P, Schmidt H, Hammerstingl C, et al. Patients with atrial fibrillation and dense spontaneous echo contrast at high risk a prospective and serial follow-up over 12 months with transesophageal echocardiography and cerebral magnetic resonance imaging. Journal of the American College of Cardiology. 2005;**45**:1807

[37] Magnani JW, Hylek EM, Apovian CM. Obesity begets atrial fibrillation: A contemporary summary. Circulation. 2013;**128**:401-405 [PubMed: 23877062]

[38] Pathak RK, Middeldorp ME, Lau DH, Mehta AB, Mahajan R, Twomey D, et al. Aggressive risk factor reduction study for atrial fibrillation

and implications for the outcome of ablation: The ARREST-AF cohort study. Journal of the American College of Cardiology. 2014;**64**:2222-2231 [PubMed: 25456757]

[39] Lip GY. Does atrial fibrillation confer a hypercoagulable state? Lancet. 1995;**346**:1313

[40] Lip GY, Lowe GD, Metcalfe MJ, et al. Effects of warfarin therapy on plasma fibrinogen, von Willebrand factor, and fibrin D-dimer in left ventricular dysfunction secondary to coronary artery disease with and without aneurysms. The American Journal of Cardiology. 1995;**76**:453

[41] Vene N, Mavri A, Kosmelj K, Stegnar M. High D-dimer levels predict cardiovascular events in patients with chronic atrial fibrillation during oral anticoagulant therapy. Thrombosis and Haemostasis. 2003;**90**:1163

[42] Sadanaga T, Sadanaga M, Ogawa S. Evidence that D-dimer levels predict subsequent thromboembolic and cardiovascular events in patients with atrial fibrillation during oral anticoagulant therapy. Journal of the American College of Cardiology. 2010;**55**:2225

[43] Goldsmith I, Kumar P, Carter P, et al. Atrial endocardial changes in mitral valve disease: A scanning electron microscopy study. American Heart Journal. 2000;**140**:777

[44] Conway DS, Pearce LA, Chin BS, et al. Plasma von Willebrand factor and soluble p-selectin as indices of endothelial damage and platelet activation in 1321 patients with nonvalvular atrial fibrillation: Relationship to stroke risk factors. Circulation. 2002;**106**:1962

[45] Conway DS, Pearce LA, Chin BS, et al. Prognostic value of plasma von Willebrand factor and soluble P-selectin as indices of endothelial damage and

platelet activation in 994 patients with nonvalvular atrial fibrillation. Circulation. 2003;**107**:3141

[46] Freestone B, Lip GY, Chong AY, et al. Circulating endothelial cells in atrial fibrillation with and without acute cardiovascular disease. Thrombosis and Haemostasis. 2005;**94**:702

[47] Boos CJ, Anderson RA, Lip GY. Is atrial fibrillation an inflammatory disorder? European Heart Journal. 2006;**27**:136

[48] Conway DS, Buggins P, Hughes E, Lip GY. Relationship of interleukin-6 and C-reactive protein to the prothrombotic state in chronic atrial fibrillation. Journal of the American College of Cardiology. 2004;**43**:2075

[49] Lip GY, Patel JV, Hughes E, Hart RG. High-sensitivity C-reactive protein and soluble CD40 ligand as indices of inflammation and platelet activation in 880 patients with nonvalvular atrial fibrillation: Relationship to stroke risk factors, stroke risk stratification schema, and prognosis. Stroke. 2007;**38**:1229

[50] Sohara H, Amitani S, Kurose M, Miyahara K. Atrial fibrillation activates platelets and coagulation in a time-dependent manner: A study in patients with paroxysmal atrial fibrillation. Journal of the American College of Cardiology. 1997;**29**:106

[51] Lip GY, Lowe GD, Rumley A, Dunn FG. Fibrinogen and fibrin D-dimer levels in paroxysmal atrial fibrillation: Evidence for intermediate elevated levels of intravascular thrombogenesis. American Heart Journal. 1996;**131**:724

[52] O'Neill PG, Puleo PR, Bolli R, Rokey R. Return of atrial mechanical function following electrical conversion of atrial dysrhythmias. American Heart Journal. 1990;**120**:353

[53] Asakura H, Hifumi S, Jokaji H, et al. Prothrombin fragment F1 + 2 and thrombin-antithrombin III complex are useful markers of the hypercoagulable state in atrial fibrillation. Blood Coagulation & Fibrinolysis. 1992;**3**:469

[54] Abe, Y, Kim, et al. Evidence for the intravascular hyperclotting state induced by atrial fibrillation itself (abstract). Journal of the American College of Cardiology 1996; 27(Suppl A):35A.

[55] Manning WJ, Silverman DI, Katz SE, et al. Impaired left atrial mechanical function after cardioversion: Relation to the duration of atrial fibrillation. Journal of the American College of Cardiology. 1994;**23**:1535

[56] Berger M, Schweitzer P. Timing of thromboembolic events after electrical cardioversion of atrial fibrillation or flutter: A retrospective analysis. The American Journal of Cardiology. 1998;**82**:1545

[57] Gentile F, Elhendy A, Khandheria BK, et al. Safety of electrical cardioversion in patients with atrial fibrillation. Mayo Clinic Proceedings. 2002;**77**:897

[58] Loh E, Sutton MS, Wun CC, et al. Ventricular dysfunction and the risk of stroke after myocardial infarction. The New England Journal of Medicine. 1997;**336**:251

[59] Chung I, Lip GY. Platelets and heart failure. European Heart Journal. 2006;**27**:2623

[60] Lip GY. Hypercoagulability and haemodynamic abnormalities in atrial fibrillation. Heart. 1997;**77**:395

[61] Blackshear JL, Pearce LA, Asinger RW, et al. Mitral regurgitation associated with reduced thromboembolic events in high-risk patients with nonrheumatic atrial fibrillation. Stroke prevention in atrial fibrillation Investigators. The American Journal of Cardiology. 1993;**72**:840

[62] Boiten J, Lodder J. Lacunar infarcts. Pathogenesis and validity of the clinical syndromes. Stroke. 1991;**22**:1374-1378 [PubMed: 1750044]

[63] Anderson DC, Kappelle LJ, Eliasziw M, et al. Occurrence of hemispheric and retinal ischemia in atrial fibrillation compared with carotid stenosis. Stroke. 2002;**33**:1963

[64] Harrison MJ, Marshall J. Atrial fibrillation, TIAs and completed strokes. Stroke. 1984;**15**:441

[65] Rovira A, Grivé E, Rovira A, Alvarez-Sabin J. Distribution territories and causative mechanisms of ischemic stroke. European Radiology. 2005;**15**(3):416-426. [Epub 19 January 2005]

[66] Lin HJ, Wolf PA, Kelly-Hayes M, et al. Stroke severity in atrial fibrillation. The Framingham Study. Stroke. 1996;**27**:1760

[67] Lamassa M, Di Carlo A, Pracucci G, et al. Characteristics, outcome, and care of stroke associated with atrial fibrillation in Europe: Data from a multicenter multinational hospital-based registry (the European Community stroke project). Stroke. 2001;**32**:392

[68] Ezekowitz MD, James KE, Nazarian SM, et al. Silent cerebral infarction in patients with nonrheumatic atrial fibrillation. The veterans affairs stroke prevention in nonrheumatic atrial fibrillation Investigators. Circulation. 1995;**92**:2178

[69] Cullinane M, Wainwright R, Brown A, et al. Asymptomatic embolization in subjects with atrial fibrillation not taking anticoagulants: A prospective study. Stroke. 1998;**29**:1810

[70] Flaker GC, Belew K, Beckman K, Vidaillet H, Kron J, Safford R, et al. Asymptomatic atrial fibrillation: Demographic features and prognostic information from the atrial fibrillation. Follow-up investigation of rhythm management (AFFIRM) study. American Heart Journal. 2005;**149**:657-663. DOI: 10.1016/j.ahj.2004.06.032

[71] Lubitz SA, Yin X, McManus DD, Weng L-C, Aparicio HJ, Walkey AJ, et al. Stroke as the initial manifestation of atrial fibrillation: The Framingham Heart study. Stroke. 2017;**48**:490-492. DOI: 10.1161/STROKEAHA.116.015071

[72] Borowsky LH, Regan S, Chang Y, Ayres A, Greenberg SM, Singer DE. First diagnosis of atrial fibrillation at the time of stroke. Cerebrovascular Diseases. 2017;**43**:192-199. DOI: 10.1159/000457809

[73] Chen PS, Chen LS, Fishbein MC, Lin SF, Nattel S. Role of the autonomic nervous system in atrial fibrillation: Pathophysiology and therapy. Circulation Research. 2014;**114**:1500-1515 [PubMed: 24763467]

[74] Gonzalez Toledo ME, Klein FR, Riccio PM, Cassara FP, Munoz Giacomelli F, Racosta JM, et al. Atrial fibrillation detected after acute ischemic stroke: Evidence supporting the neurogenic hypothesis. Journal of Stroke and Cerebrovascular Diseases. 2013;**22**:e486-e491 [PubMed: 23800494]

[75] Berge E, Whiteley W, Audebert H, De Marchis GM, Fonseca AC, Padiglioni C, et al. European Stroke Organisation (ESO) guidelines on intravenous thrombolysis for acute ischaemic stroke. European Stroke Journal. 2021;**6**(1):I-LXII

[76] National Institute of Neurological Disorders and Stroke rt-PA Stroke Study Group. Tissue plasminogen activator for acute ischemic stroke. The New England Journal of Medicine. 1995;**333**:1581

[77] Hart RG, Palacio S, Pearce LA. Atrial fibrillation, stroke, and acute antithrombotic therapy: Analysis of

randomized clinical trials. Stroke. 2002;**33**:2722

[78] Sposato LA, Cipriano LE, Saposnik G, Ru z Vargas E, Riccio PM, Hachinski V. Diagnosis of atrial fibrillation after stroke and transient ischaemic attack: A systematic review and meta-analysis. Lancet Neurology. 2015;**14**:377-387. DOI: 10.1016/S1474-4422(15)70027-X

[79] European Stroke Organisation (ESO) Executive Committee; ESO Writing Committee. Guidelines for management of ischaemic stroke and transient ischaemic attack 2008. Cerebrovascular Diseases. 2008;**25**: 457-507. DOI: 10.1159/000131083

[80] Jauch EC, Saver JL, Adams HP Jr, Bruno A, Connors JJ, Demaerschalk BM, et al. Guidelines for the early management of patients with acute ischemic stroke: A guideline for healthcare professionals from the American Heart Association/American Stroke Association. Stroke. 2013;**44**:870-947. DOI: 10.1161/STR.0b013e318284056a

[81] Kernan WN, Ovbiagele B, Black HR, Bravata DM, Chimowitz MI, Ezekowitz MD, et al. Guidelines for the prevention of stroke in patients with stroke and transient ischemic attack: A guideline for healthcare professionals from the American Heart Association/American Stroke Association. Stroke. 2014;**45**:2160-2236. DOI: 10.1161/STR.0000000000000024

[82] Kirchhof P, Benussi S, Kotecha D, Ahlsson A, Atar D, Casadei B, et al. 2016 ESC guidelines for the management of atrial fibrillation developed in collaboration with EACTS. European Heart Journal. 2016;**37**:2893-2962. DOI: 10.1093/eurheartj/ehw210

[83] Aguilar MI, Hart R, Pearce LA. Oral anticoagulants versus antiplatelet therapy for preventing stroke in patients with non-valvular atrial fibrillation and no history of stroke or transient ischemic attacks. Cochrane Database of Systematic Reviews. 2007; **18**(3): CD006186 Jul 18;(3)

[84] van Walraven C, Hart RG, Singer DE, et al. Oral anticoagulants vs aspirin in nonvalvular atrial fibrillation: An individual patient meta-analysis. Journal of the American Medical Association. 2002;**288**:2441-2448

[85] Ogilvie IM, Welner SA, Cowell W, et al. Ischaemic stroke and bleeding rates in 'real-world' atrial fibrillation patients. Thrombosis and Haemostasis. 2011;**106**:34-44

[86] NICE. Available at: www.nice.org.uk. In: Atrial Fibrillation: The Management of Atrial Fibrillation. NICE; 2014 National Clinical Guideline Centre (UK). London, UK: National Institute for Health and Care Excellence; 2014 Jun

[87] European Heart Rhythm A, European Association for Cardio-Thoracic S, Camm AJ, et al. Guidelines for the management of atrial fibrillation: The task force for the management of Atrial fibrillation of the European Society of Cardiology (ESC). Europace. 2010;**12**:1360-1420

[88] Stroke Prevention in Atrial Fibrillation Study. Final results. Circulation. 1991;**84**:527

[89] Warfarin versus aspirin for prevention of thromboembolism in atrial fibrillation: Stroke prevention in Atrial fibrillation II study. Lancet. 1994;**343**:687

[90] Petersen P, Boysen G, Godtfredsen J, et al. Placebo-controlled, randomised trial of warfarin and aspirin for prevention of thromboembolic complications in chronic atrial fibrillation. The Copenhagen AFASAK study. Lancet. 1989;**1**:175

[91] Ezekowitz MD, Bridgers SL, James KE, et al. Warfarin in the prevention of stroke associated with nonrheumatic atrial fibrillation. Veterans affairs stroke prevention in nonrheumatic atrial fibrillation investigators. The New England Journal of Medicine. 1992;**327**:1406

[92] Connolly SJ, Laupacis A, Gent M, et al. Canadian Atrial Fibrillation Anticoagulation (CAFA) study. Journal of the American College of Cardiology. 1991;**18**:349

[93] Risk factors for stroke and efficacy of antithrombotic therapy in atrial fibrillation. Analysis of pooled data from five randomized controlled trials. Archives of Internal Medicine. 1994;**154**:1449

[94] Cooper NJ, Sutton AJ, Lu G, Khunti K. Mixed comparison of stroke prevention treatments in individuals with nonrheumatic atrial fibrillation. Archives of Internal Medicine. 2006;**166**:1269

[95] McNamara RL, Tamariz LJ, Segal JB, Bass EB. Management of atrial fibrillation: Review of the evidence for the role of pharmacologic therapy, electrical cardioversion, and echocardiography. Annals of Internal Medicine. 2003;**139**:1018

[96] Hylek EM, Go AS, Chang Y, et al. Effect of intensity of oral anticoagulation on stroke severity and mortality in atrial fibrillation. The New England Journal of Medicine. 2003;**349**:1019

[97] Lip GY, Nieuwlaat R, Pisters R, et al. Refining clinical risk stratification for predicting stroke and thromboembolism in atrial fibrillation using a novel risk factor-based approach: The euro heart survey on atrial fibrillation. Chest. 2010;**137**:263-272

[98] Pisters R, Lane DA, Nieuwlaat R, et al. A novel user-friendly score

(HAS-BLED) to assess 1-year risk of major bleeding in patients with atrial fibrillation: The Euro Heart survey. Chest. 2010;**138**:1093-1100

[99] Connolly SJ, Eikelboom J, Joyner C, et al. Apixaban in patients with atrial fibrillation. The New England Journal of Medicine. 2011;**364**:806-817

[100] Connolly SJ, Ezekowitz MD, Yusuf S, et al. Dabigatran versus warfarin in patients with atrial fibrillation. The New England Journal of Medicine. 2009;**361**:1139-1151

[101] Patel MR, Mahaffey KW, Garg J, et al. Rivaroxaban versus warfarin in nonvalvular atrial fibrillation. The New England Journal of Medicine. 2011;**365**: 883-891

[102] Giugliano RP, Ruff CT, Braunwald E, et al. Edoxaban versus warfarin in patients with atrial fibrillation. The New England Journal of Medicine. 2013;**369**:2093-2104

[103] Holbrook AM, Pereira JA, Labiris R, et al. Systematic over- view of warfarin and its drug and food interactions. Archives of Internal Medicine. 2005;**165**:1095-1106

[104] Aithal GP, Day CP, Kesteven PJ, et al. Association of poly-morphisms in the cytochrome P450 CYP2C9 with warfarin dose requirement and risk of bleeding complications. Lancet. 1999;**353**:717-719

[105] D'Andrea G, D'Ambrosio RL, Di Perna P, et al. A polymorphism in the VKORC1 gene is associated with an interindividual variability in the dose-anticoagulant effect of warfarin. Blood. 2005;**105**:645-649

[106] Husted S, de Caterina R, Andreotti F, et al. Non-vitamin K antagonist oral anticoagulants (NOACs): no longer new or novel. The Journal of Thrombosis and Haemostasis. 2014;**111**:781-782. 29

[107] Yeh CH, Fredenburgh JC, Weitz JI. Oral direct factor Xa inhibitors. Circulation Research. 2012;**111**: 1069-1078

[108] Lee CJ, Ansell JE. Direct thrombin inhibitors. British Journal of Clinical Pharmacology. 2011;**72**:581-592

[109] Granger CB, Alexander JH, McMurray JJ, et al. Apixaban versus warfarin in patients with atrial fibrillation. The New England Journal of Medicine. 2011;**365**:981

[110] Alexander JH, Wojdyla D, Vora AN, et al. Risk/benefit Tradeoff of antithrombotic therapy in patients with Atrial fibrillation early and late after an acute coronary syndrome or percutaneous coronary intervention: Insights from AUGUSTUS. Circulation. 2020;**141**:1618

[111] Okumura K, Akao M, Yoshida T, et al. Low-dose edoxaban in very elderly patients with atrial fibrillation. The New England Journal of Medicine. 2020;**383**:1735

[112] Lip GY, Skjøth F, Rasmussen LH, Larsen TB. Oral anticoagulation, aspirin, or no therapy in patients with nonvalvular AF with 0 or 1 stroke risk factor based on the CHA2DS2-VASc score. Journal of the American College of Cardiology. 2015;**65**:1385

[113] Lip GYH, Banerjee A, Boriani G, et al. Antithrombotic therapy for Atrial fibrillation: CHEST guideline and expert panel report. Chest. 2018;**154**:1121

[114] Borre ED, Goode A, Raitz G, et al. Predicting thromboembolic and bleeding event risk in patients with non-valvular Atrial fibrillation: A systematic review. Thrombosis and Haemostasis. 2018;**118**:2171

[115] Friberg L, Rosenqvist M, Lip GY. Net clinical benefit of warfarin in patients with atrial fibrillation: A report from the Swedish atrial fibrillation cohort study. Circulation. 2012;**125**:2298

[116] Singer DE, Chang Y, Fang MC, et al. The net clinical benefit of warfarin anticoagulation in atrial fibrillation. Annals of Internal Medicine. 2009;**151**:297

[117] Olesen JB, Lip GY, Lindhardsen J, et al. Risks of thromboembolism and bleeding with thromboprophylaxis in patients with atrial fibrillation: A net clinical benefit analysis using a 'real world' nationwide cohort study. Thrombosis and Haemostasis. 2011;**106**:739

[118] Banerjee A, Lane DA, Torp-Pedersen C, Lip GY. Net clinical benefit of new oral anticoagulants (dabigatran, rivaroxaban, apixaban) versus no treatment in a 'real world' atrial fibrillation population: A modelling analysis based on a nationwide cohort study. Thrombosis and Haemostasis. 2012;**107**:584

[119] Lee CJ, Toft-Petersen AP, Ozenne B, et al. Assessing absolute stroke risk in patients with atrial fibrillation using a risk factor-based approach. The European Heart Journal - Cardiovascular Pharmacotherapy. 2021;**7**:f3

[120] Ganesan AN, Chew DP, Hartshorne T, Selvanayagam JB, Aylward PE, Sanders P, et al. The impact of atrial fibrillation type on the risk of thromboembolism, mortality, and bleeding: A systematic review and meta-analysis. European Heart Journal. 2016;**37**:1591-1602. DOI: 10.1093/ eurheartj/ehw007

[121] Hess PL, Healey JS, Granger CB, Connolly SJ, Ziegler PD, Alexander JH, et al. The role of cardiovascular implantable electronic devices in the detection and treatment of subclinical atrial fibrillation: A review. JAMA Cardiology. 2017;**2**:324-331. DOI: 10.1001/jamacardio.2016.5167

[122] Thijs V. Atrial fibrillation detection. Fishing for an irregular heartbeat before and after stroke. Stroke. 2017;**48**:2671-2677

[123] Van Gelder IC, Healey JS, Crijns HJGM, Wang J, Hohnloser SH, Gold MR, et al. Duration of device-detected subclinical atrial fibrillation and occurrence of stroke in ASSERT. European Heart Journal. 2017;**38**:1339-1344. DOI: 10.1093/eurheartj/ehx042

[124] Diederichsen SZ, Haugan KJ, Brandes A, et al. Natural history of subclinical atrial fibrillation detected by implanted loop recorders. Journal of the American College of Cardiology. 2019;**74**:2771

[125] Kezerle L, Tsadok MA, Akriv A, et al. Pre-diabetes increases stroke risk in patients with nonvalvular atrial fibrillation. Journal of the American College of Cardiology. 2021;**77**:875

[126] Lubitz SA, Yin X, Rienstra M, Schnabel RB, Walkey AJ, Magnani JW, et al. Long-term outcomes of secondary atrial fibrillation in the community: The Framingham Heart study. Circulation. 2015;**131**:1648-1655. DOI: 10.1161/CIRCULATIONAHA.114.014058

[127] Gialdini G, Nearing K, Bhave PD, Bonuccelli U, Iadecola C, Healey JS, et al. Perioperative atrial fibrillation and the long-term risk of ischemic stroke. Journal of the American Medical Association. 2014;**312**:616-622. DOI: 10.1001/jama.2014.9143

[128] Ahlsson A, Fengsrud E, Bodin L, Englund A. Postoperative atrial fibrillation in patients undergoing aortocoronary bypass surgery carries an eightfold risk of future atrial fibrillation and a doubled cardiovascular mortality. European Journal of Cardio-Thoracic Surgery. 2010;**37**:1353-1359. DOI: 10.1016/j. ejcts.2009.12.033

[129] Lowres N, Mulcahy G, Gallagher R, Ben Freedman S, Marshman D,

Kirkness A, et al. Self-monitoring for atrial fibrillation recurrence in the discharge period post-cardiac surgery using an iPhone electrocardiogram. European Journal of Cardio-Thoracic Surgery. 2016;**50**:44-51. DOI: 10.1093/ejcts/ezv486

[130] Guo Y, Lane DA, Chen Y, et al. Regular bleeding risk assessment associated with reduction in bleeding outcomes: The mAFA-II randomized trial. The American Journal of Medicine. 2020;**133**:1195

[131] Poli D, Antonucci E, Grifoni E, et al. Bleeding risk during oral anticoagulation in atrial fibrillation patients older than 80 years. Journal of the American College of Cardiology. 2009;**54**:999

[132] Fang MC, Go AS, Chang Y, et al. Death and disability from warfarin-associated intracranial and extracranial hemorrhages. The American Journal of Medicine. 2007;**120**:700

[133] Ruff CT, Giugliano RP, Braunwald E, et al. Comparison of the efficacy and safety of new oral anticoagulants with warfarin in patients with atrial fibrillation: A meta-analysis of randomised trials. Lancet. 2014;**383**:955-962

[134] ACTIVE Writing Group of the ACTIVE Investigators, Connolly S, Pogue J, et al. Clopidogrel plus aspirin versus oral anticoagulation for atrial fibrillation in the Atrial Fibrillation Clopidogrel Trial with Irbesartan for prevention of Vascular Events (ACTIVE W): A randomised controlled trial. Lancet. 2006;**367**:1903

[135] ACTIVE Investigators, Connolly SJ, Pogue J, et al. Effect of clopidogrel added to aspirin in patients with atrial fibrillation. The New England Journal of Medicine. 2009;**360**:2066

[136] Tereshchenko LG, Henrikson CA, Cigarroa J, Steinberg JS. Comparative

effectiveness of interventions for stroke prevention in atrial fibrillation: A network meta-analysis. Journal of the American Heart Association. 2016;**5**: 1-17

[137] Själander S, Själander A, Svensson PJ, Friberg L. Atrial fibrillation patients do not benefit from acetylsalicylic acid. Europace. 2014;**16**:631

[138] Adjusted-dose warfarin versus low-intensity. Fixed-dose warfarin plus aspirin for high-risk patients with atrial fibrillation: Stroke prevention in atrial fibrillation III randomised clinical trial. Lancet. 1996;**348**:633

[139] Gulløv AL, Koefoed BG, Petersen P, et al. Fixed minidose warfarin and aspirin alone and in combination vs adjusted-dose warfarin for stroke prevention in atrial fibrillation: Second Copenhagen atrial fibrillation, aspirin, and anticoagulation study. Archives of Internal Medicine. 1998;**158**:1513

[140] Paciaroni M, Agnelli G, Ageno W, Caso V. Timing of anticoagulation therapy in patients with acute ischaemic stroke and atrial fibrillation. Thrombosis and Haemostasis. 2016;**116**:410

[141] Chen ZM, Sandercock P, Pan HC, et al. Indications for early aspirin use in acute ischemic stroke : A combined analysis of 40 000 randomized patients from the chinese acute stroke trial and the international stroke trial. On behalf of the CAST and IST collaborative groups. Stroke. 2000;**31**:1240

[142] Gomez-Outes A, Terleira-Fernandez AI, Calvo-Rojas G, et al. Dabigatran, rivaroxaban, or apixaban versus warfarin in patients with nonvalvular atrial fibrillation: A systematic review and meta-analysis of subgroups. Thrombosis. 2013;**2013**: 640723

[143] Chao TF, Liu CJ, Lin YJ, et al. Oral anticoagulation in very elderly patients with atrial fibrillation: A nationwide cohort study. Circulation. 2018;**138**:37

Chapter 4

Atrial Cardiopathy and Cryptogenic Stroke

Marianela López Armaretti, Natalia Romina Balian and María Cristina Zurrú

Abstract

Cryptogenic stroke (CS) is defined as the presence of cerebral infarcts, the cause which has not been identified despite an appropriate diagnostic evaluation, and it accounts for approximately 30–40% of all ischemic strokes. There is a certain subgroup of CS with embolic characteristics on neuroimaging studies and no evidence of atrial fibrillation alternative or any alternative cause. Recent data suggest that disorders of the atrium, even without atrial fibrillation, could increase thromboembolic risk. The pathological atrial substrate, or atrial cardiopathy (AC), may be an important and underrecognized cause of cryptogenic strokes. This chapter will review the information on the rationale and data behind the concept of atrial cardiopathy, its pathophysiology, proposed biomarkers of atrial cardiopathy, and therapeutic implications.

Keywords: cryptogenic stroke, atrial fibrillation, atrial cardiopathy, atrial disease, atrial dysfunction

1. Introduction

Cryptogenic stroke (CS) can be defined as the presence of cerebral infarcts, the cause of which has not been identified after an appropriate diagnostic evaluation is performed, and it accounts for approximately 30–40% of all ischemic strokes.

To define an ischemic event as cryptogenic, four conditions must be excluded: (1) small deep infarcts in the distribution of penetrating cerebral vessels (<15 mm on CT, <20 mm on MRI diffusion images); (2) intracranial or extracranial stenosis (>50% luminal stenosis of the artery supplying the ischemic area); (3) a defined cardioembolic source identified by transthoracic echocardiography or electrocardiography (ECG); or (4) certain defined entities such as vasculitis, hypercoagulability, migraine, vasospasm, and dissection [1].

There is a subgroup of CS with imaging features suggestive of a distant embolic source. Such characteristics are the presence of multiple, cortical infarcts affecting the territory of major branches of the cerebral arterial tree, with non-lacunar appearance. This subtype has been referred to as Embolic Stroke of Undetermined Source (ESUS) to describe an embolic-appearing CS [2].

Some proposed mechanisms for CS include paroxysmal atrial fibrillation (AF), patent foramen ovale, aortic arch atheroma, atherosclerosis of intracranial and extracranial vessels, hypercoagulability, and cerebral vasculitis.

Identifying the main cause of ischemic stroke is more than an academic issue since each specific stroke subtype often guides secondary stroke prevention strategies.

A novel potential cause of CS is atrial cardiopathy (AC), which involves atrial structural or functional abnormalities that may occur with AF, but also in the absence of AF. There are many CS patients with evidence suggestive of AC indicated by the presence of one of its serum, imaging, or ECG biomarkers, which could potentially explain some of these "unexplained" strokes [3].

Actually, the clinical value of identifying patients with AC is that it not only reduces diagnostic uncertainty, avoiding the need to search for other causes of stroke, but it may also have specific implications for treatment.

2. Atrial cardiopathy: rationale and biological mechanisms

AC is an emerging potential etiology of CS and refers to left atrial structural or functional disorders that may occur with AF but also in its absence. However, if an AF is diagnosed in the context of an ischemic stroke, definite cardioembolic origin is usually established unless a concurrent source is present.

The disorders of the left atrium (LA) can be congenital or acquired. Among the latter, left atrial enlargement (LAE) provides a ground for thrombus formation through stasis, inflammation, and endothelial dysfunction. The consequence may be visible with echocardiography as spontaneous echogenicity, sludge, or directly as a thrombus, all different stages of a thrombotic substrate. In addition, myocardial fibrosis may provide another mechanism for cardiac embolism. It involves the progressive accumulation of fibrotic tissue within the LA myocardium, basically related with the senescence of the heart, but also associated with acute or chronic systemic inflammation. This leads to fibrotic replacement, structural remodeling, and electrical changes, predisposing to AF [4, 5].

Among congenital disorders, certain LA morphologies as well as the size of LAA orifice are thought to increase the thromboembolic risk. A retrospective study of 932 patients with AF who were evaluated with cardiac images (CCT or CMR) categorized the left atrial appendage (LAA) into four distinct morphologies: chicken wing (48%), cactus (30%), windsock (19%), and cauliflower (3%). The prevalence of ischemic stroke among different LAA morphologies was: 4% in chicken wing, 10% in windsock, 12% in cactus, and 18% in cauliflower. Moreover, the number of trabeculations was an independent predictor of stroke risk, and in this regard, the cauliflower morphology seems to have the highest risk. In the same way, LAA flow velocity is a known inverse marker of stroke risk. This flow velocity was highest among patients with chicken wing as opposed to non-chicken-wing morphology, which may also explain why the chicken wing morphology has the lowest risk of ischemic stroke. Also, a larger LAA orifice area has been associated with ischemic stroke. Perhaps, LAA morphology can still be a predictor of thrombus generation and embolic risk even in the absence of AF [6].

Accordingly, these data compilations suggest that electrical AF does not provide the unique explanation for embolic events in patients with evidence of atrial dysfunction and that AC is an innovative factor to keep in mind.

Although the specific criteria for AC are being refined, it may be diagnosed by the presence of one of the biomarkers of left atrial dysfunction that will be detailed below.

3. Biomarkers of atrial cardiopathy

The diagnostic algorithm for AC should follow a step-by-step strategy, in which the risk factors for atrial heart disease, electrical and mechanical atrial dysfunction, and increased thrombotic risk must be identified. The markers of left atrial dysfunction can be divided into three groups:

1. Echocardiographic (enlargement, volume and/or function of the left atrium, anatomy of the left atrial appendage, and spontaneous echocardiographic contrast).

2. Electrocardiographic (increased terminal force of the P wave in V1, episodes of subclinical atrial tachyarrhythmia, atrial extrasystoles, and interatrial block).

3. Serum biomarkers (N-Terminal pro-Brain Natriuretic Peptide and highly sensitive cardiac troponin assay).

3.1 Echocardiographic biomarkers

a. Left atrial enlargement: In population-based studies, LAE has been shown to be associated with incident AF and incident ischemic stroke risk. An analysis from the Framingham study showed that LA diameter was associated with stroke risk in men and women. An analysis from the Northern Manhattan Stroke Study (NOMASS) showed an association between left atrial index and ischemic stroke. Also, this study demonstrated that moderate to severe LAE is an independent predictor of recurrent stroke risk.

b. Spontaneous echogenicity: Spontaneous echogenicity (SE) can be detected by transesophageal echocardiography, less commonly through a transthoracic view. It is an echocardiographic feature characterized by a dynamic smoke-like appearance in the left atrium or left atrial appendage and is a demonstration of blood stasis and hypercoagulability, particularly in an enlarged LA.

c. Echocardiographic markers of left atrial appendage: In sinus rhythm, the LAA is a contractile structure that empties all its contents with each beat. In atrial fibrillation, there is a loss of its contractile property with dilatation, which leads to slowed blood flow, with the consequent increase in the risk of thrombosis. Approximately 90% of the thrombi located in the left atrium are found within the appendage. In fact, recent trials of left atrial appendage closure showed that successful LAA closure was non-inferior to warfarin in reducing the risk of ischemic stroke, suggesting a functional and structural role of the LAA, greater than AF itself, in ischemic stroke risk.

As mentioned above, different LAA morphologies may also be associated with different flow velocities in the LAA, leading to different thrombosis risk levels.

Reduced LAA flow velocity on echocardiography can promote stasis and thrombus formation. In a post-hoc analysis from the Stroke Prevention in Atrial Fibrillation (SPAF)-III trial that included 721 patients who underwent TEE, a peak anterograde flow velocity of less than 20 cm/s was independently associated with thrombus formation and risk of cardio embolism.

3.2 Electrocardiogram markers

a. Paroxysmal supraventricular tachycardia: Although paroxysmal supraventricular tachycardia (PSVT) has been considered a conduction disorder arising
   mostly in young and healthy individuals, there is evidence that proposes that it
   occurs in two different populations: young patients with lone PSVT and older
   patients with cardiovascular disease. Furthermore, there are studies report-
   ing that nearly 12% of patients with PSVT develop incident AF during a 1-year
   follow-up. It seems that in certain individuals, PSTV may be a prelude of atrial
   cardiopathy.

b. Increased P-wave terminal force in V1: The P-wave terminal force in lead V1
   (PTFV1) on ECG measures the electrical conduction through the atria. Any
   disorder in atrial functioning may cause prolongation in the P-wave terminal
   force. Evidence from observational cohorts suggests that elevated PTFV1
   is associated with the risk of ischemic stroke, particularly those related to
   embolism (cryptogenic or cardioembolic) and independent of AF.

c. Others: Prolongation of the PR interval on ECG is another biomarker of atrial
   disease. There is a reported association between PR interval prolongation and
   incident AF after cryptogenic stroke. Furthermore, a recent multicentric study
   showed that a prolonged PR interval (PR ≥ 200 ms) was more prevalent in
   cryptogenic stroke.

Bayes syndrome, an arrhythmological syndrome characterized by advanced
interatrial block, is another potential biomarker of atrial cardiopathy. This
syndrome is a predictor of AF, ischemic stroke risk particularly of the cardioembolic
subtype, silent cerebrovascular disease, and vascular cognitive impairment.

3.3 Cardiac magnetic resonance imaging markers

3.3.1 Atrial fibrosis and delayed gadolinium enhancement

Cardiac MRI (CMR) has been used for cardiac disorders, but its use in
cryptogenic stroke is not well established. There is a potential role for CMR in the
diagnostic evaluation of patients with cryptogenic stroke to identify potential
etiologies such as cardiac thrombi, cardiac tumors, aortic arch disease, and other
rare cardiac anomalies. It can also provide data on certain functional and structural
parameters of the LA and the LAA associated with ischemic stroke risk. Cardiac
fibrosis can be detected on MRI as a delay in uptake of gadolinium. The relationship
between cardiac fibrosis on cardiac MRI and stroke risk remains unclear. Therefore,
studies investigating this association are needed to determine whether and to what
extent gadolinium enhancement is delayed and is associated with thromboembolic
risk in the absence of AF.

3.4 Serum biomarkers

a. NT-proBNP: N-Terminal pro-Brain Natriuretic Peptide (NTpro-BNP) is a serum
   biomarker of cardiac disease that partly reflects atrial myocyte dysfunction. An
   elevated NTpro-BNP level is a marker of cardiac dysfunction and stretch, volume overload, and a predictor of cardiovascular events including incident AF.
   Studies have shown an association between elevated NT-proBNP and ischemic

stroke, particularly of the embolic subtype. In fact, a post-hoc analysis of the WARSS trial showed a reduction in the risk of stroke or death at 2 years among those patients with the highest NT-proBNP values (> 750 pg./ml) assigned to warfarin rather than aspirin.

b. HS cTnT: Cardiac troponin (cTnT) is another serum biomarker of cardiac injury, often used to determine the presence of cardiac ischemia. A highly sensitive (hs) cTnT assay can detect concentrations more than 10 times lower than conventional assays used for the detection of acute cardiac ischemia. HS cTnT is associated with the risk of cardiovascular events in observational studies. In the ARIC study (n = 10.902, mean follow up 11.3 years), the highest quintile showed an association between hs cTnT and ischemic stroke risk but not between HS cTnT and non-lacunar strokes. Therefore, HS cTnT is another serum biomarker of cardiac injury that is associated with embolic stroke subtypes [7–9].

4. Therapeutic implications

Patients with atrial cardiopathy and cryptogenic stroke may benefit from anticoagulation therapy for secondary stroke prevention. Anticoagulation therapy has been shown to reduce stroke risk in certain cardiac disorders. In patients with AF, anticoagulation with warfarin or a novel oral anticoagulant is associated with at least 50% reduction in risk of stroke or systemic embolism.

Warfarin also reduces the risk of ischemic stroke in patients with mechanical heart valves and in those with left ventricular thrombus after anterior myocardial infarction.

Given that most cardiac thrombi in patients with AF arise in the left atrium/left atrial appendage, and since anticoagulation is effective in reducing the risk of cardiac thrombi, it is possible that patients with AC and CS constitute another group of patients who may benefit from anticoagulation therapy.

To date, AF is the only marker of left atrial dysfunction for which anticoagulation has been shown to provide a greater reduction of stroke risk than antiplatelet therapy.

Additional trials testing the efficacy of anticoagulant therapy in individuals with markers of AC are required.

The ongoing ATTICUS and ARCADIA trials are trying to validate this hypothesis, and the results may have implications for secondary stroke prevention as well as primary prevention. If anticoagulant therapy demonstrates a reduction in recurrent stroke in the AC high-risk population, it may be beneficial for patients with AC and no history of stroke [3, 10, 11].

5. Conclusions

The key to prevention of stroke is understanding its cause. AC, as determined by the presence of biomarkers of left atrial dysfunction, may constitute one of the mechanisms beyond CS, and validation of this concept would allow a therapeutic strategy to be implemented not only in secondary but also in primary prevention. Awaiting the occurrence or detection of AF in CS patients with AC may expose them to another event, so clinical trials testing anticoagulation versus antiplatelet therapy to reduce stroke risk are needed and welcome.

6. Key points

- AC may be defined as a functional or structural disorder of the left atrium.

- Biomarkers of atrial dysfunction or cardiopathy have been associated with a risk of first and recurrent ischemic stroke, particularly those related to embolism.

- Up to one-third of ischemic strokes are currently cryptogenic. Approximately 65% of CS patients have AC, as evidenced by at least one of its biomarkers.

- 70% of CS patients do not have AF, even after 3 years of cardiac monitoring. This indicates that AF may not be the only necessary substrate for cardio embolism.

- Patients with AC and CS may benefit from anticoagulation therapy for secondary stroke prevention, and ongoing trials are underway.

Author details

Marianela López Armaretti*, Natalia Romina Balian and María Cristina Zurrú
Hospital Italiano of Buenos Aires, Argentina

*Address all correspondence to: marianela.lopez@hospitalitaliano.org.ar

IntechOpen

References

[1] Yaghi S, Kamel H, Elkind MSV. Atrial cardiopathy: A mechanism of cryptogenic stroke. Expert Review of Cardiovascular Therapy. 2017;**15**(8): 591-599

[2] Jalini S, Rajalingam R, Nisenbaum R, Javier AD, Woo A, Pikula A. Atrial cardiopathy in patients with embolic strokes of unknown source and other stroke etiologies. Neurology. 2019;**92**(4): e288-e294

[3] Kamel H, Longstreth WT Jr, Tirschwell DL, Kronmal RA, Broderick JP, Palesch YY, et al. The Atrial cardiopathy and antithrombotic drugs in prevention after cryptogenic stroke randomized trial: Rationale and methods. International Journal of Stroke. 2019;**14**(2):207-214

[4] Leifer D, Rundek T. Atrial cardiopathy: A new cause for stroke? Neurology. 2019;**92**(4):155-156

[5] Elkind MSV. Atrial Cardiopathy and stroke prevention. Current Cardiology Reports. 2018;**20**(11):103

[6] Gwak DS, Choi W, Kim YW, Kim YS, Hwang YH. Impact of left atrial appendage morphology on recurrence in embolic stroke of undetermined source and atrial cardiopathy. Frontiers in Neurology. 2021;**22**(12):679320

[7] Yaghi S, Boehme AK, Hazan R, Hod EA, Canaan A, Andrews HF, et al. Atrial cardiopathy and cryptogenic stroke: A cross-sectional pilot study. Journal of Stroke and Cerebrovascular Diseases. 2016;**25**(1):110-114

[8] Edwards JD, Healey JS, Fang J, Yip K, Gladstone DJ. Atrial cardiopathy in the absence of atrial fibrillation increases risk of ischemic stroke, incident atrial fibrillation, and mortality and improves stroke risk prediction. Journal of the American Heart Association. 2020;**9**(11):e013227

[9] Chen J, Gao F, Liu W. Atrial cardiopathy in embolic stroke of undetermined source. Brain and Behavior: A Cognitive Neuroscience Perspective. 2021;**11**(6):e02160

[10] Hart RG, Sharma M, Mundl H, Kasner SE, Bangdiwala SI, Berkowitz SD, et al. Rivaroxaban for stroke prevention after embolic stroke of undetermined source. The New England Journal of Medicine. 2018;**378**:2191-2201

[11] Diener HC, Sacco RL, Donald Easton J, Granger CB, Bernstein RA, Uchiyama S, et al. Dabigatran for prevention of stroke after embolic stroke of undetermined source. The New England Journal of Medicine. 2019;**380**:1906-1917

Chapter 5

Vascular Brain Disease in Geriatric Neuropsychiatry

Gilberto Sousa Alves and Felipe Kenji Sudo

Abstract

Vascular brain diseases are a significant cause of dementia, and their presence, alone or associated with degenerative conditions, increases the risk of conversion to progressive cognitive decline. Neuropsychiatric manifestations vary according to the affected brain territory and disrupted neuronal circuits. In the current chapter, epidemiological prevalence, the harmonization of the diagnostic criteria of vascular subtypes, and the impact of age and socio-demographic aspects are critically reviewed. Another explored topic refers to the diagnostic and therapeutic approach. Structural imaging, including magnetic resonance (MRI) and computer tomography (CT), and a thorough neuropsychological and clinical exam, may help establish the differential diagnosis and substantially impact clinical evolution. Treatment involves various strategies, including controlling cardiovascular and metabolic risk factors, such as hypertension, atrial fibrillation, cardiopathies, and adopting a healthy lifestyle. Treatment relies on preventive and health promotion strategies related to the timely control of vascular risk factors and symptomatic approaches. The use of acetylcholinesterase inhibitors aims at stabilizing symptoms and is recommended in all stages of dementia.

Keywords: brain, vascular, cognitive impairment, geriatric neuropsychiatry

1. Introduction

The concept of vascular dementia (VaD) is a diagnostic category that emerged in the late 1980s to characterize dementia secondary to cerebrovascular disease [1]. The construct was later expanded into the Vascular Cognitive Involvement complex (VCI), a continuum ranging from Vascular Mild Cognitive Impairment (VMCI) to dementia [2]. This chapter will comprehensively address the main clinical, diagnostic, and therapeutic aspects of VCI.

2. Epidemiology

2.1 Population studies

Recent studies estimated that between 5 and 7% of the world's elderly population suffers from dementia, with a higher frequency in Latin America (8.5%) and a slightly lower prevalence in sub-Saharan Africa (2–4%) [3]. Considering the high social and economic impact of the condition, especially in these regions with fast population aging, knowledge of the epidemiology of dementia has become fundamental for planning health policies [4, 5].

From an etiological point of view, cerebrovascular disease is the second most common cause of acquired cognitive impairment and dementia, occurring both as a single mechanism of brain damage and contributing to cognitive decline in neuro-degenerative dementias [6]. Cerebral arteriosclerosis was considered the leading cause of "senile dementia" until the 1960s when Alzheimer's Disease (AD) became recognized as the most prevalent brain pathology affecting those individuals [7, 8]. Recently, cognitive impairment of vascular origin has once again attracted the interest of researchers, driven mainly by the growing concern with metabolic conditions (systemic arterial hypertension, diabetes mellitus, dyslipidemia and obesity) and their effects on target organs [9, 10]. The incidence rate of dementia appears to be declining in western developed countries, which has been hypothesized to result from continued improvements in older adult education and advances in health care, including efficiently controlling metabolic diseases [11, 12].

Challenges for understanding and interpreting the epidemiological aspects of VCI to include the lack of harmonization of the nomenclature and diagnostic criteria used in the studies. **Table 1** lists some of the primary population studies produced between 2000 and 2012, which have estimated the prevalence of VaD in different countries. A meta-analysis reported that VaD occurs in 1.6% of individuals over 65 years of age and constitutes 26% of the total number of people with dementia in western countries [13]. Conflicting results across studies could be identified, mostly derived from different sources of diagnostic criteria employed: when the National Institute of Neurological Disorders and Stroke and *l'Association Internationale pour la Recherche et l'Enseigne* (NINDS-AIREN) criteria was adopted, the prevalence of VaD was 1.6%; conversely, the adoption of Alzheimer's Disease Diagnostic and Treatment Centers (ADDTC) criteria yielded a prevalence of 2.6% [4].

2.2 Brain vascular changes and cognition

One study demonstrated that 83.3% of individuals with dementia due to subcortical vascular disease initially presented focal or mild changes in cognition, with low impact on functionality, which would be analogous to the concept of Mild Cognitive Impairment due to AD [14]. Vascular Cognitive Impairment non Dementia, another construct of prodromal VaD, presented a prevalence of 2.6–8.5% in samples older than 65, configuring the most common clinical form among VCI cases [15].

In addition to etiological characteristics, other aspects may impact the prevalence of VaD in studies, such as age and geographic aspects, i.e., the inclusion of populations from long-term care facilities and the presence of comorbid brain conditions with neurodegenerative processes. Some studies demonstrated an increase in VaD prevalence with aging, although lesser than that observed in AD. It was suggested that the prevalence of VaD would double every 5.3 years, while AD would present a prevalence twice as high every 4.3 years [6]. Consistently, prevalence rates below 1% were identified in some studies that included samples younger than 65 years of age, whereas in a study evaluating a 95-year-old group, the prevalence was 15.7% (**Table 1**). However, conflicting results could be found in the literature on the relationship between aging and VaD. A European study, for example, showed that the prevalence of VaD reduced when populations aged 60 and 90 were compared—15 and 8.7%, respectively [16]. In addition, the variation in the prevalence of VaD between the eighth and tenth decades of life was not significant in one study (from 10.2 to 9.9%) [16, 17]. Mixed dementia, on the other hand, showed that prevalence between these age groups increased, advancing from 4.7 to 7.1% of subjects [16, 17]. Another study conducted in the USA showed that VaD was responsible for 21% of dementia cases among those 80 years of age, but this rate corresponded to only 16% of cases older than 80. Studies evaluating the prevalence

Country	Author, year	Sample (n)	Diagnostic criteria	Age (years)	Prevalence
China	Wang W et al., 2000	3728	DSM-III-R, ICD-10	≥65	1.37%
	Zhang ZX et al., 2005	34807	MINDS-AIREN	≥65	1.1%
	Zhao Q et al., 2010	17018	DSM-IV, NINDS-AIREN	≥55	0.79%
	Jia J et al., 2014	10276	DSM-IV, NINDS-AIREN	≥65	0.79%
South Korea	Lee DY et al., 2002	643	DSM-IV	≥65	2%
	Jhoo JH et al., 2008	1118	DSM-IV, NINDS-AIREN	≥65	1%
	Kim KW et al., 2011	8199	DSM-IV, NINDS-AIREN	≥65	2%
Japan	Yamada T et al., 2001.	3715	DSM-III-R, NINDS-AIREN	≥65	1%
	Ikeda M et al., 2001	1162	DSM-IV	≥65	2.4%
	Meguro K et al., 2002	1654	DSM-IV, ADDTC, NINDS-AIREN	≥65	1.6% (NINDS-AIREN) and 2.6% (ADDTC)
	Wada-Isoe K et al., 2009	120	DSM-IV, NINDS-AIREN	≥65	1.7%
Thailand	Wangtongkum S et al., 2008.	1492	DSM-IV, NINDS-AIREN	≥45	0.29%
Sri Lanka	de Silva HA et al., 2003	703	DSM-IV	≥65	0.57%
Turkey	Arslantaş D, Ozbabalik D, 2009	3100	CID-10	≥55	4.29%
Spain	Vilalta-Franch J et al., 2000	1460	CAMDEN	≥70	6.23%
	García García et al., 2001	3214	DSM-III-R, NINDS-AIREN	≥65	1.8%
	Bofill E et al., 2009	877	DSM-IV, NINDS-AIREN	≥80	6%
Denmark	Andersen K et al., 2000	3346	DSM-III-R	65–84	1.3%
Sweden	Börjesson-Hanson A et al., 2004	338	DSM-III-R	95	15.7%
USA	Plassman BL et al., 2007	856	DSM-III-R, DSM-IV	≥71	2.43%
Brazil	Herrera Jr. et al., 2002	1656	NINDS-AIREN.	≥65	0.66%
	Bottino CM et al., 2008	1563	DSM-IV	≥60	2%
Egypt	The Callaway HN et al., 2012	8173	DSM-IV-TR	≥50	0.64%

Table 1.
Population studies of VAD prevalence.

of early-onset dementia (starting before 65 years old) have also documented controversial results. VaD was shown to be the leading cause of early-onset dementia in a Japanese retrospective study, affecting 42.5% of the cases [18], while a Spanish study, which evaluated the incidence of dementia in individuals aged 30–64 years, reported that VaD was responsible for only 13.8% of cases; therefore, occurring less frequently than AD (42.4%) and dementia secondary to general medical conditions (18.1%) [19].

Geographic issues may affect the prevalence of VaD across studies. Classical studies have recorded the high prevalence of VaD in Japan and China, which would account for 50% of dementia cases, overcoming the frequency of AD [13]. Recent studies, however, have not confirmed such findings. It is currently accepted that, as observed in other countries, AD is the most common etiology of dementia in these regions. Meguro et al. [20] have argued that epidemiological studies previously conducted in Japan had overestimated the occurrence of VaD, probably due to categorizing mixed dementia within the group with cerebrovascular-related cognitive impairments [4]. Consequently, VaD/AD prevalence ratios significantly decreased in individuals 75 years old or more in studies conducted in Japan from 1985 to 2005 (2.1 in 1985; 1.2 in 1992; 0.7 in 1998 and 0.7 in 2005) [21]. In Brazil, the prevalence of VaD ranged from 9.3 to 15.9% of dementia cases in population studies conducted in São Paulo state [22–24]. Studies evaluating differences between regions with different degrees of urbanization reported controversial results. The overall prevalence of dementia in rural areas of China was significantly higher than in urban areas (6.05% vs. 4.40%, P < 0.001), but this difference was not observed for VaD (1.28% vs. 1.61%, P = 0.166) [25]. Other authors, however, suggested that living in rural areas would double the odds of developing VAD (odds-ratio = 2.03) [26].

Comorbidity between AD and vascular brain lesions seems frequent. *Postmortem* studies indicated that 34% of individuals who presented pathological brain markers of AD also suffered from vascular brain changes [27]. Likewise, another article showed that significant vascular abnormalities occurred in 89% of cases of AD [28]. A population study reported that 40% of patients with dementia presented a combination of AD-related and vascular brain alterations [4]. However, few studies to date have evaluated the prevalence of mixed dementia. A study showed that 12.6% of dementia cases met diagnostic criteria for both AD and VaD [29].

Studies measuring the influence of gender on the prevalence of VaD also produced conflicting results. Moreover, systemic arterial hypertension may double the risk for VaD in females, but not in males, while physical exercises appear to protect women more efficiently than men from VaD [26].

Studies on the incidence of VaD are rare and conflicting in the literature. According to North American data, VaD, with or without associated AD component, has an annual incidence of 14.6 per 1000 people for Caucasians and 27.2 per 1000 people for African Americans [30]. According to studies, the incidence rates of VaD did not differ between men and women [27].

3. Classification and diagnosis

3.1 Subtypes and clinical criterium

Cognitive alterations due to cerebrovascular disease (CVD) have been classified within a continuum named Vascular Cognitive Impairment (VCI), and the term VaD is currently reserved for the stages in which such deficits reach dementia severity [2, 31]. The concept of VCI involves presymptomatic presentations with high risk for cerebrovascular disease ("brain-at-risk"), as well as cases of cognitive impairment of vascular etiology that do not meet criteria for VaD, referred to as Vascular Cognitive Impairment No-Dementia (V-CIND) or Vascular Mild Cognitive Impairment (VaMCI) [6, 32].

VCI encompasses a combination of various types of cerebral vascular lesions, i.e., multiple cortical or subcortical infarctions, strategic infarctions, microangiopathic lesions of white matter, base nuclei hypoperfusion lesions, and hemorrhagic lesions [31]. As a result of the array of pathological processes leading to parenchymal damage, heterogeneous clinical presentations, including motor, cognitive and neuropsychiatric manifestations, could be identified. Hence, to enable a didactic approach to these conditions, some authors have sought to define VCI subsyndromes based on the mechanism of vascular brain injury, which generated the concepts of "dementia by multiple infarctions," "dementia by strategic infarction," and "vascular dementia by subcortical ischemia."

Dementia due to multiple infarctions results from disease of the large cerebral vessels, resulting mainly from vascular thromboembolism. Cortico-subcortical infarctions of variable extension are observed [33]. Symptoms typically start abruptly and evolve in a stepwise pattern, succeeding ischemic brain events. With the accumulation of brain lesions, the patient begins to develop focal neurological signs, such as asymmetric reflexes, pseudobulbar syndrome (i.e., difficulties swallowing and speaking, in addition to effective lability), the release of primitive reflexes (such as Babinski reflex), and sensory abnormalities [33].

Dementia by strategic infarction is understood as a single lesion (or few lesions), which occurs in a functionally important location. It may result from cortical or subcortical infarction, whether unilateral or bilateral. Examples are dementias resulting from thalamic or hippocampal infarction [33].

Dementia due to subcortical ischemic vascular disease (SIVD) is the most frequent subtype of VaD, and it is associated with changes in small cerebral vessels (perforating arteries) disease, secondary mainly to hypertensive arteriopathy. It covers two clinical subsyndromes: Binswanger disease and lacunar state. Binswanger disease consists of dementia due to large subcortical infarctions, while in lacunar infarcts, multiple punctiform or rounded lesions are observed in the cerebral parenchyma. The clinical picture is usually insidious in most cases.

VaD due to subcortical ischemia may also be associated with the presence of a mutation in the NOTCH3 gene, of autosomal dominant transmission, causing the disease known by the acronym CADASIL (cerebral autosomal dominant arteriopathy with subcortical infarcts and leukoencephalopathy). This disorder presents as VaD by multiple subcortical infarctions of presenile onset. Symptoms include, in addition to severe cognitive deficits, the presence of migraine with aura, mood swings, and apathy.

The most used diagnostic guidelines for the detection of VaD are summarized in **Table 2**. Except for Hachinski's Ischemic Score (HIS), based solely on clinical criteria, the diagnosis of VAD depends on the demonstration of cognitive deficits through neuropsychological testing and the relationship between cognitive impairment and the vascular brain alterations identified to neuroimaging. The definition of dementia varies according to the criteria employed, leading to difficulties interpreting the results of studies that use different diagnostic systems.

3.2 Historical evolution of the VCI concept

Although the evolution of knowledge about the clinical and neuroimaging characteristics of VCI has led to the improvement of diagnostic guidelines, some questions remain. The HIS, elaborated in 1975, was one of the first instruments to suggest a differentiation between "dementia by multiple vascular infarctions" and "primary degenerative dementia" through clinical criteria. Among them, the items "abrupt onset" and "stepwise evolution" refer to the pattern of cognitive deficits that follow episodes of vascular ischemia (e.g., vascular brain ictus). Following this principle,

Diagnostic criteria	EIH (1975)	ADDTC (1992)	CID-10 (1992)	NINDS-AIREN (1993)	ASA/AHA (2011)	DSM-5 (2013)
Clinical criteria	Abrupt onset, "stepwise" evolution, fluctuation, nocturnal confusion, personality preservation, depression, somatic complaints, emotional lability, arterial hypertension, history of stroke, focal symptoms, focal signs, other signs of arteriosclerosis	Cognitive decline in more than one domain, CVD (demonstrated by a history of two or more vascular events, focal neurological signs, or one stroke with a clear temporal relationship with cognitive alterations), functional impairment, high HIS, history of TIAs, history of risk factors for CVD (hypertension, diabetes, heart disease)	Impairment of memory and intellectual activities (thinking, reasoning, and flow of ideas), with consequent functional impairment, absence of disturbance of consciousness, deterioration of emotional control, social behavior and motivation, focal neurological signs, deficits present for at least six months.	Memory impairment +1 other cognitive domain, functional impairment, focal signs, the onset of dementia up to 3 months after stroke, abrupt onset, fluctuating course or "stepwise progression," other signs suggestive of CVD (gait disorders, falls, change in urinary frequency or urgency, pseudobulbar paralysis, abulia, depression, emotional incontinence, psychomotor retardation, executive dysfunction)	Impairment in two or more cognitive domains demonstrated by tests, functional impairment; a clear temporal relationship between deficits and vascular event or a clear relationship between severity and pattern of cognitive impairment; the presence of subcortical and diffuse CVD, absence of progressive evolution of deficits suggestive of neurodegenerative disorder	The onset of symptoms related to one or more vascular brain events, evidence of a more prominent decline in attention (including processing speed) and executive function, CVD by history, physical examination, and neuroimaging
Laboratory criteria/ neuroimaging	—	Evidence of 2 or more areas of vascular lesions at neuroimaging, evidence of at least one vascular lesion (in non-cerebellar location), presence of multiple infarctions	Presence of cortical, subcortical, or mixed infarctions	Evidence of CVD to neuroimaging, two or more ischemic events, severe territorial, strategic, or subcortical infarction	Evidence of CVD to neuroimaging	Evidence of CVD to a degree sufficient to cause cognitive symptoms, significant brain parenchyma injury, genetic evidence of CVD

Table 2.
Diagnostic criteria for vascular dementia.

more recent diagnostic guidelines require a temporal relationship between vascular events and cognitive impairment. However, recognizing subcortical ischemic disease as a cause of dementia of insidious evolution makes it necessary to adapt the criteria for the best detection of this type of condition. In addition, the memory impairment requirement, present in ICD-10 and NINDS-AIREN, derives from an approximation between VaD and more specific cognitive attributes of AD. The DSM-5, published in 2013, has brought advances in this aspect, highlighting the presence of compromises in attention, processing speed, and executive function. Another data that deserves attention is the inaccuracy of neuroimaging criteria since the extent of white matter lesions necessary to generate cognitive alterations with dementia severity is not defined by the classification systems. Finally, the requirement of deficits in at least two domains is consensual among the most recent diagnostic guidelines. However, the cut-off point for cognitive impairment is not established. The National Institutes of Health (NIH) defined the cognitive impairment due to dementia as a cognitive performance of two standard deviations below normative data in at least two cognitive domains, albeit further studies are needed to evaluate the validity of these criteria.

Predementia cognitive alterations of vascular etiology began to draw the attention of researchers in the late 1990s when Bowler's studies warned of the importance of an early diagnosis for VCI [31]. Although the authors already pointed to the need for new diagnostic criteria that included the initial stages of the condition, early studies with Mild Cognitive Impairment (MCI) sought their similarities with AD [34]. In 2003, a study group meeting in Stockholm expanded the concept of MCI to include the "non-amnesic" form of the disorder in the diagnostic criteria [34]. Petersen's diagnostic guidelines published in 2004 placed the MCI as a risk factor for dementia of different etiologies. In vascular conditions, amnestic or non-amnestic MCI with multi-domain involvement would tend to progress to VaD [34]. However, this initial model only included cognitive and functional aspects, not defining neuroimaging criteria for the condition. In 2011, the diagnostic criteria for VMCI were published, developed by the American Heart Association and the American Stroke Association, inspired by the algorithm for detecting VaD proposed by these same entities [6]. The Vascular Cognitive Impairment No-Dementia (VCIND) construct is a more comprehensive concept than the VMCI, since it encompasses a wide range of conditions affecting cognition in the late life, including focal cognitive deficits, genetic disorders, and cognitive alterations secondary to psychiatric disorders. However, a review of the concept of VCIND, proposed by Zhao et al. restricted this construct to bring it closer to the concept of VMCI [35]. The DSM-5 established the diagnostic guidelines for the Mild Neurocognitive Disorder of vascular etiology, defining it as the presence of subtle cognitive impairments due to cerebrovascular disease [36].

Dementia associated with multiple mechanisms of brain damage, such as vascular-related and neurodegenerative processes, has been classified as Mixed Dementia (MD). Despite its increasing prevalence, the concept of MD lacks a clear definition. The HIS conceptualizes MD as an intermediate clinical state with both VaD and AD characteristics [33]. The NINDS-AIREN (1993) did not establish diagnostic criteria for DM, recommending the term "AD + Cerebrovascular disease" [37]. ICD-10 proposed that the diagnosis of MD should be established if the subject fulfilled the criteria for both AD and VaD [38]. The DSM-5 does not present a diagnosis characterization of DM but indicates the possibility of a simultaneous diagnosis of VAD and AD [36].

In addition, diagnostic definitions of VCI generally require observing cognitive dysfunction, vascular risk factors, vascular brain lesions, and focal neurological findings [39]. A classic presentation with stepwise evolution can be found in large-vessel disease [33]. **Table 3** summarizes these aspects.

	Risk and etiological factors	Age of onset	Neuroimaging	Clinical features
Multi-infarct	Hypertension, heart disease, diabetes, coronary disease	From the 4th decade	Cortical lesions and/or white matter and basal ganglia; commitment of the anterior, posterior and middle cerebral arteries	Executive dysfunction, apathy, impairment in attention depression, psychomotor slowing
CADASIL	Mutation of the NOCHT 3 gene	3–4th decades	Hyperintensities in the temporal subcortical region	Migraine, executive dysfunction, family history
Binswanger	Age, hypertension, diabetes	Between 4 and 7th decades	Extensive and diffuse lesions in the subcortical region	Insidious progression, mood swings, psychomotor slowing apathy, motor changes
Lacunar infarctions	Cardiac arrhythmias (atrial fibrillation), heart disease, hypertension	From the 4th decade. Present in up to 30% of individuals over 30 years of age	Lesions in areas adjacent to the lateral ventricles, basal ganglia, thalamus, inner capsule, bridge, and cerebellum	"Silent infarctions"; the presence of risk factors, varied clinical and related to the topography of lesions.

Table 3.
Clinical and radiological features of VaD.

4. Pathophysiology

4.1 Cardiovascular aspects related to VaD

Hypoperfusion related to atherosclerosis and arterial sclerosis, hypotension associated with reduced cholinergic activity, altered autonomic regulation, cortical hypometabolism, disruption of the neurovascular unit, and cardiovascular events such as congestive heart failure, with consequent systolic dysfunction and embolism is among the main events related to cerebrovascular disease and cognitive decline [6, 40]. Vascular lesions may cause impairment in cholinergic function and disconnection of frontal limbic associative fibers. Cholinergic tracts integrate different brain areas, participating in vasomotor control and cognitive and behavioral modulation [33].

SIVD is commonly observed in MRI in the form of subcortical hyperintensities. It results from the interplay of multiple risk factors affecting cerebral small vessels, such as dyslipidemia, hypertension, heart disease, genetics, and diabetes mellitus. Microstructural abnormalities usually comprise gliosis, demyelination, and axonal damage of subcortical connections. White matter lesions, known as leukoaraiosis, may be related to apathy, executive dysfunction, depression, motor alterations, and urinary control and have been considered a reliable predictor for progression to dementia [41]. Studies have shown that extensive white matter lesions, characterized by a score equal to 3 on the Fazekas visual scale, may have a death or disability rate of 29.5%. On the other hand, the identification of leukoaraiosis at MRI may not be exclusively suggestive of SIVD. Additional pathological processes, including inflammation (e.g., multiple sclerosis and neurosarcoidosis), autoimmune diseases (celiac disease), and inherited metabolism errors (leukodystrophy), may appear hyperintense at neuroimaging.

Metabolic	Cardiovascular	Lifestyle	Others
High cholesterol	Arterial hypertension	Tobacco smoking	Psychological stress
Diabetes mellitus	Arteriosclerosis	Alcoholism	Depression
Metabolic syndrome	Atrial fibrillation	Sedentarism	Sleep apnea
High homocysteine	Coronary disease	Inadequate diet	Low education
Obesity	Carotid stenosis		Heart surgery
	Myocardial inflammation		Vasculitis
	Valvulopathy		
	Patent foramen ovale		

Table 4.
Modifiable vascular risk factors.

Cognitive impairment resulting from SIVD may increase the risk for conversion into dementia and directly cause cognitive decline. Executive dysfunction, attention deficit, processing slowing, and visuospatial alterations are frequently observed [36]. Memory impairment tends to be less severe than AD, as it mainly affects free recall and usually spares recognition, and patients can benefit from clues. Apathy, depression, and anxiety are standard features of SIVD. Possibly, a relationship between the extent of the lesions and the location exists with the severity of dementia.

Binswanger disease is characterized as damage of 25% or more of the subcortical region [42]. It is characterized pathologically by thickening the walls of the small arteries with fibrinoid necrosis of large caliber brain vessels [43].

4.2 Vascular risk factors

Vascular risk factors (VRF) encompass disorders with an increased chance of developing brain vessel pathology and circulatory disorders, with eventual nervous tissue damage (CVD), leading to CCV14 [44].

The VRF comprises various causes (genetic, metabolic, cardiovascular, lifestyle, others) underlying the vascular pathology and eventually the nervous tissue supplied by the vascular territory. They can be divided into non-modifiable, currently without adequate treatment or prevention (e.g., genetic [cerebral amyloid angiopathy, CADASIL, Fabry disease]) and modifiable, i.e., amenable to treatment and prevention (e.g., metabolic, cardiovascular) [45–47] (**Table 4**). The various VRF, including genetic diseases, and vascular pathologies, such as embolisms, cerebral blood flow, and perfusional changes, must be considered.

5. Diagnosis

5.1 Clinical evaluation and complementary exams

Anamnesis should investigate vascular risk factors, including arterial hypertension, dyslipidemia, diabetes mellitus, and sickle cell anemia [33]. Previous personal or familial history of vascular brain events should be characterized. Lifestyle habits, including alcohol and tobacco consumption and unhealthy diet, are strongly associated with VCI.

Clinical evaluation should also be directed to screening cognitive symptoms, especially to difficulties for goal-directed behaviors and sustained attention, as well as for deficits in cognitive speed [36]. Other abnormalities may include problems remembering recent events, difficulties organizing the personal agenda and planning tasks, reduced verbal fluency, and impaired spatial orientation.

Behavioral changes, either sudden or insidious, such as irritability, reduced general interest, and social isolation, often indicate depressive symptoms. In addition, personality changes, visible in social situations where the behavioral pattern is beyond the usual, may denote changes in brain function. A third component aspect of anamnesis is functional assessment, which addresses the degree of autonomy for resolving indoor or outdoor tasks, such as making a meal, paying bills, or dealing with money. For greater diagnostic accuracy, it is always desirable to have a companion throughout the examination, preferably those with recurrent or continuous contact, considering the possibility of cognitive impairment in the patient.

The detailed neurological clinical examination should be guided by investigating comorbidities such as hypertension, atrial fibrillation, dehydration, infection, delirium, number of prescribed medications, alteration of sphincter control, motor difficulties or speech articulation, the occurrence of falls, as sudden changes in the level of consciousness.

5.2 Neuropsychological assessment

The neuropsychological and clinical characteristics of VaD vary depending on the location and extent of the lesions. Neuropsychological evaluation analyzes the repercussions of brain lesions and dysfunctions on the cognition and behavior of the patient [48]. The differential diagnosis of AD and VaD, the most frequent types of dementia, can be challenging; as previously mentioned, those two pathological processes may share similar clinical characteristics, and they may co-occur [1]. In addition, neuropsychological evaluation may help assess clinical status, contributing to planning therapeutic strategies and family guidance [49]. Some of the main findings on neuropsychological differences in the most homogeneous group of SIVD and AD are summarized in **Table 5**.

5.3 Neuroimaging assessment

Different guidelines recommend the use of neuroimaging for the characterization of cerebrovascular disease [6, 39, 50–53]. Initially, as proposed by the National Institute of Neurological Disorders and Stroke–Canadian Stroke Network in 2006, these methods were recommended solely in research settings [50]. In 2011, with the American Heart Association/American Stroke Association recommendations, neuroimaging became a critical diagnostic tool in clinical practice [6].

Cognitive function	SIVD	AD
Memory	• Minor impairment of episodic memory; Relative preservation of recognition memory, with benefit in the face of recognition clues	• Marked impairment in episodic memory (immediate memory and evocation); little benefit in the face of recognition clues
Language	• More significant impairment in phonemic verbal fluency; • Lower frequency of naming errors	• More significant impairment in semantic verbal fluency; • Higher frequency of naming errors
Executive functions	• Marked impairment in planning tests, "sequencing," cognitive flexibility, and alternating attention; • Impairment in psychomotor speed	• Improved performance in executive function tests and psychomotor speed

Table 5.
Differential diagnosis of VAD and AD according to cognition.

5.3.1 Structural brain neuroimaging

Computed tomography (CT) is sufficient to rule out other causes of cognitive decline besides VCI, such as tumor processes, subdural hematoma, or hydrocephalus. Lacunar infarctions and, to a lesser extent, subcortical lesions can be seen on CT. The detection of vascular brain disease by magnetic resonance imaging (MRI) is made through T2 and Flair-weighted images (**Figures 1** and **2**), the latter being the preferred sequence for identifying subcortical hyperintensities. In the case of thalamic strategic infarctions, the T2 sequence can contribute to its more precise location. Micro bleeds and calcifications may be better detected with the use of T2-weighted images. The finding of watershed infarcts between the anterior and middle cerebral artery is usually seen in the dominant hemisphere, in the case of anterior cerebral artery flow territories, bilaterally, preferably by FLAIR sequences.

The presence of lesions suggestive of ischemia or lacunar infarction on MRI or tomography should always be correlated with clinical examination and neuropsychological examination findings. On the other hand, the absence of vascular lesions on CT or MRI indicates the low probability of a vascular etiology of dementia. The operational guidelines of the NINDS-AIREN - Association Internationale pour la Recherche et l'Enseignement en Neurosciences - are used to understand the radiological aspects of VCI, being fundamental for the diagnosis of probable VaD [33, 37].

Subcortical vascular lesions result from small vessel disease and can be identified at MRI as pointy, diffuse, or localized areas, hyperintense in FLAIR and T2-weighted sequences [53]. Some authors distinguished their locations in periventricular and subcortical. Several studies in neuroimaging have adopted volumetric techniques for the measurement of neuroimaging volume. However, visual methods have wide use in the clinical routine, giving their straightforward interpretation an advantage. One is the use of the Fazekas scale (**Figure 1**), ranging from 0 to 3. Recommendations for neuroimaging characterization of SIVD also include the analyses of cerebral microbleeds and perivascular spaces [39, 50, 53].

Diffusion tensor or diffusion tensor imaging (DTI) is a structural resonance technique based on the displacement of water molecules along axon fibers. DTI can be very useful as a biological marker of loss of axonal integrity and is a promising technique in the early diagnosis of neuronal disconnections in several neuropsychiatric conditions, including VAD. Studies investigating brain vascular-related changes have shown the importance of evaluating specific brain regions, such as

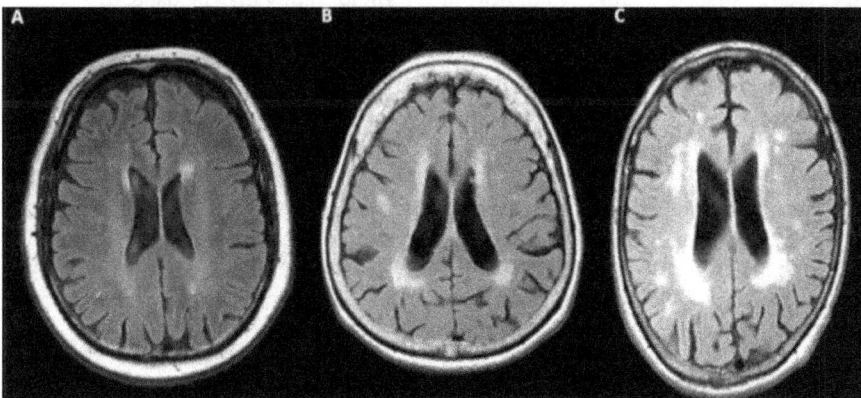

Figure 1.
The proportion of white matter hyperintensities to magnetic resonance imaging with FLAIR sequence. The score on the Visual Scale of Fazekas for light (A), moderate (B), and advanced (C) levels were corresponding to the score of 1, 2, and 3, respectively.

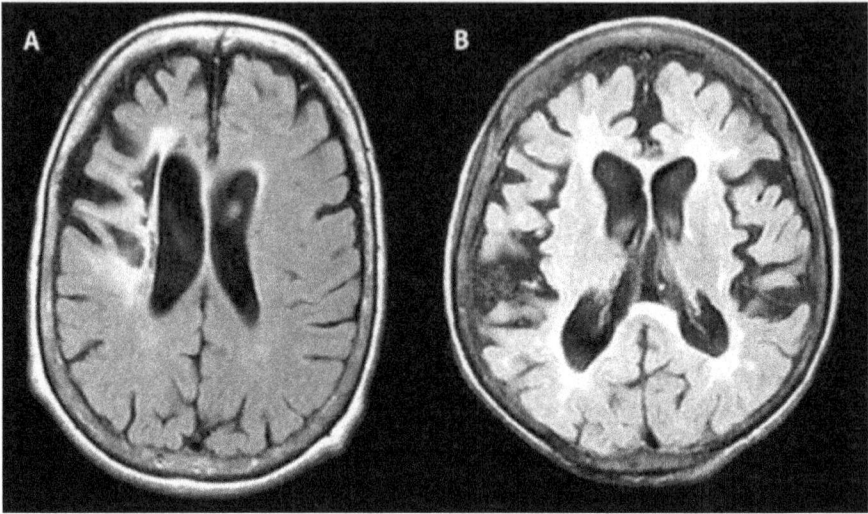

Figure 2.
Flair image (A) shows cortico-subcortical infarction on the right, corresponding to the anterior cerebral artery territory with caudate nucleus injury. In some individuals, extensive white matter injury correlates with more significant overall cortical atrophy and increased risk for dementia, as shown in image (B).

fornix, cingulate, and hippocampus; another focus of clinical interest of DTI has been the investigation between vascular and degenerative factors in dementia, especially the role of ischemic vascular lesions in conversion to AD [54]. In addition, axonal lesions may be associated with increased blood pressure, even in the absence of a diagnosis of hypertension [55].

5.3.2 Structural imaging in peripheric vascular disease

Neurovascular evaluation includes several complementary tests, such as ultrasonography (USG) of cervical carotid and vertebral arteries and CT or RM angiography of the carotid and vertebral arteries. These tests investigate vascular pathologies, e.g., atheromatous plaques and changes in cerebral blood flow. In cases where detailed visualization of the cervical and intracranial arterial tree is necessary, such as suspected aneurysm, MRI or CT angiography may be used.

5.3.3 Perfusion and molecular methods

The use of single-photon emission tomography (SPECT) seems relevant in the differential diagnosis with VAD and, in typical Binswanger-type VaD, the finding of diffuse hypoperfusion. Concerning positron emission tomography (PET), different patterns of metabolism reduction are usually associated with VAD; these include diffuse hypometabolism in SIVD, frontal or multifocal, as in the case of lacunar or multiple infarctions. The use of PET or SPECT is recommended in the investigation of atypical cases, in which there are doubt diagnoses after clinical examination and structural neuroimaging.

5.4 Behavioral assessment

The comorbidity of VCI and mood disturbances, particularly affective symptoms, led to the proposition of a hypothesis known as "vascular depression" [56]. Statistically, anxiety (70%) and depression (20%) are the most frequent symptoms found in VCI [57]. Studies estimate that the prevalence of depression in VaD is 13.1% in community samples and 21.4% in-hospital samples [57]. The high prevalence of depression in VAD (8–66%) and the frequent occurrence of visual hallucinations, especially in multi-infarct dementia, were observed compared to AD [58]. Conversely, mania (1%), psychotic symptoms are less common but have frequency similar to that encountered in AD.

The neuropathological mechanisms associated with behavioral alterations result from frontal and or subcortical involvement in different circuits and may reflect diffuse lesions or strategic anatomical structures. Behavioral changes may be accompanied by cognitive symptoms, such as concentration difficulties, slowing cognitive processing, and executive dysfunction.

6. Treatment principles

6.1 General principles of treatment

Considering the absence of specific treatment of CCV, the available therapeutic strategies comprise, above all, aspects of prevention [45, 59]. Therefore, the binomial control of risk factors—promotion of good health constitutes the main objective from the individual, epidemiological and public health point of view. Successful prevention depends on the control and modification of risk factors and the effectiveness of protective factors, such as adequate lifestyle (including diet, physical activity, among others) [46]. It should be emphasized that prevention measures should be maintained from the brain-at-risk to the various CCV symptomatic presentations.

Neuropsychiatric symptoms are seen in all phases of CCV, most marked in the more advanced ones. Its treatment is necessary, considering its interference in other areas of performance and the quality of life of patients and family members. Treatment can be established after the correct definition of the problem, away from personal environmental factors of discomfort, and the differential diagnosis (e.g., delirium [infectious, metabolic, or drug-induced confusional states]). Initially, non-pharmacological strategies (environmental, behavioral, psychological, should be used) and pharmacological treatment, when indicated, should be safe and effective, minimizing cardiovascular side effects to avoid additional vascular injury [60].

The treatment of VaD can be didactically divided into pharmacological and non-pharmacological strategies. The first includes preventive measures based on epidemiological findings, e.g., the effective control of vascular risk factors [61]. Therefore, there is consensus among the authors regarding the need to treat hypertension, dyslipidemia, diabetes, and other associated factors, although the effect size of preventive, therapeutic interventions for each risk factor remains disputable [6]. Nevertheless, studies suggest that effective control of hypertension results in a decrease of up to 34% in the incidence of VaD.

6.2 Non-pharmacological treatment

6.2.1 Control of cardiovascular and metabolic risk factors

Both hypertension and diabetes and have been related to the higher incidence of VCI. Blood glucose control should be moderate (glycated hemoglobin between 7 and 7.9%); however, scarce evidence for a specific class of antihypertensive drugs remains [6, 62]. Patients with heart disease, e.g., atrial fibrillation, should be carefully monitored for appropriate anticoagulation levels. Smoking cessation should be stimulated regardless of age group.

6.2.2 Physical exercise

Evidence from animal studies points to the benefits of physical activity in angio-genesis, brain, and neurogenesis. Population studies have confirmed these findings by demonstrating a favorable role of physical activity in the lowest conversion rate for dementia and the most beneficial evolution [6]. However, the benefits seem less robust for VaD than for AD [6].

6.2.3 Diet and supplementation

The higher intake of polyunsaturated acids and omega 3, fibers, bowls of cereal, the moderate consumption of milk and its derivatives, meats, and saturated fatty acids have been associated with reducing the conversion of MCI and AD. Moderate alcohol use in about one or two drinks (<30 g/d) and adequate weight control also had a protective effect on VAD development. The mechanisms underlying this effect would be reducing LDL, increased HDL, reducing alcohol consumption, insulin resistance and blood pressure, reducing platelet aggregation and serum fibrinogen and homocysteine levels and inflammatory markers.

6.2.4 Neuropsychological rehabilitation

Neuropsychological rehabilitation may have a role in the treatment of cognitive deficits and neuropsychiatric symptoms in VCI. Individual or group family support can also be valuable in the rehabilitation process, providing caretakers with infor-mation about the disease and prognosis and offering emotional support for coping [63]. Most studies with cognitive intervention, however, showed reduced efficacy in improving cognitive function with cognitive rehabilitation. Some findings highlight the lack of evidence due to methodological difficulties, such as the duration of the intervention, the instruments used as the control of confounding variables (medi-cal comorbidities and psychiatric alterations).

6.3 Pharmacological treatment

6.3.1 The use of cholinesterase inhibitors

The frequent overlap of pathological mechanisms between VaD and AD sug-gests that the use of acetylcholinesterase inhibitors may be useful in patients with vascular brain disease. The use of donepezil showed good tolerability and may improve cognitive and functional status. Rivastigmine has shown to be effective on cognition, although with an effect size proportionally lower than donepezil [62].

The use of cholinesterase inhibitors and the N-methyl-D-aspartate (NMDA) receptor modulators in patients with VaD and VCI has been controversial, although the benefits seem more evident with specific groups, e.g., individuals with the subcortical disease. Memantine, an NMDA antagonist, would act on the toxic action caused by glutamatergic overactivation, putatively exhibiting brain neuroprotective properties. There is also a need for further evidence demonstrating the benefits of this medication in VAD, but some specialists point to a possible improvement in subcortical conditions [62].

6.3.2 Treatment of behavioral changes in VCI

Pharmacological treatment of behavioral alterations aims at symptomatic remission or stabilization. Antidepressants may be indicated in moderate or severe depressive symptoms or when monotherapy with acetylcholinesterase inhibitors has no effective response. Serotonin reuptake inhibitors (SSRI), venlafaxine, mirtazapine, and trazodone are usually regarded as the safest and most well-tolerated options.

The use of trazodone or anticonvulsant has been used in maniform symptoms, agitation, or aggressive behavior. Carbamazepine shows evidence of success in reducing agitation. Newer drugs such as gabapentin may still show effectiveness in these conditions. Atypical antipsychotics may also be an alternative in agitation, and use should be restricted to the acute period. Risperidone and olanzapine are drugs with better tolerability. However, the occurrence of sedation and risk and falls and the evidence of increased incidence of drug-related vascular events demand thorough dosage monitoring, with the risks and benefits being weighed on a case-by-case basis.

6.3.3 Alternative treatments

The use of ginkgo Biloba, nimodipine (potassium channel blocker), and antioxidant agents requires further scientific evidence.

Regarding surgical interventions, studies have sought evidence of improvement in cognitive function after carotid revascularization, but the results are still inconclusive. Conversely, studies have pointed to cognitive improvement after carotid stent implantation against embolism, but these results require confirmation with long-term follow-up of patients.

7. Conclusion

This chapter provided a concise review of epidemiological, diagnostic, and clinical aspects of vascular brain diseases. For most countries, vascular brain disease is a significant cause of dementia, and their presence, alone or associated with degenerative conditions, increases the risk of conversion to progressive cognitive decline. Neuropsychiatric manifestations vary according to the affected brain territory and disrupted neuronal circuits; behavioral disturbances include, for instance, mood, psychomotor, or thought disorders; cognitive deficits involve memory, attention, language, and other alterations, depending on the extension and localization of the lesions. Early diagnosis may have a decisive impact on clinical evolution and should guide health policies involving the old age population. Treatment involves a wide range of strategies, including controlling cardiovascular and metabolic risk factors and adopting a healthy lifestyle. Pharmacological treatment may include cholinesterase inhibitors and NMDA modulators, which aim to stabilize symptoms and, although not officially approved, are recommended depending on the stages of dementia. The safety and effectiveness of antipsychotics and antidepressants, particularly in managing agitation, psychosis, and depression, require further studies.

Conflict of interests

The authors declare no conflict of interests.

Abbreviations

AD	Alzheimer's dementia
TIA	transient ischemic attack
CADASIL	cerebral autosomal dominant arteriopathy with subcortical infarcts and leukoencephalopathy

CVD	cerebrovascular disorders
DTI	diffusion tensor imaging
HIS	Hachinski ischemic scale
HIE	hemorrhagic ischemic events
ICD	international classification of diseases
MCI	mild cognitive impairment
MD	mixed dementia
NINDS-AIREN	Association Internationale pour la Recherche et l'Enseignement en Neurosciences
NMDA	N-methyl-D-aspartate
VaD	vascular dementia
VCI	vascular cognitive impairment
VCIND	vascular cognitive impairment not dementia
VMCI	mild cognitive impairment of vascular origin
VRF	vascular risk factors
SIVD	subcortical vascular ischemic disease
SPECT	single-photon emission tomography

Author details

Gilberto Sousa Alves[1,2*†] and Felipe Kenji Sudo[3]

1 Translational Research Group in Psychiatry, Federal University of Maranhão, São Luís, Maranhão, Brazil

2 Post Graduation in Psychiatry and Mental Health, PROPSAM, Federal University of Rio de Janeiro, Rio de Janeiro, Brazil

3 D'Or Institute for Research and Education, Rio de Janeiro, RJ, Brazil

*Address all correspondence to: gsalves123@hotmail.com

† All authors contributed equally.

IntechOpen

References

[1] Román G. Diagnosis of vascular dementia and Alzheimer's disease. International Journal of Clinical Practice. Supplement. 2001;**120**:9-13

[2] Hachinski V. Vascular dementia: A radical redefinition. Dementia and Geriatric Cognitive Disorders. 1994;**5**(3-4):130-132

[3] Prince M, Albanese E, Guerchet M, Prina M. World Alzheimer Report 2014. Dementia and Risk Reduction. An Analysis of Protective and Modifiable Factors [Internet]. Alzheimer's Disease International (ADI); 2014. Available from: https://www.alzint.org/u/WorldAlzheimerReport2014.pdf

[4] Meguro K, Ishii H, Yamaguchi S, Ishizaki J, Shimada M, Sato M, et al. Prevalence of dementia and dementing diseases in Japan: The Tajiri project. Archives of Neurology. 2002;**59**(7):1109

[5] Prince M, Wimo A, Guerchet M, Ali G-C, Wu Y-T, Prina M, Alzheimer's Association. World Alzheimer Report 2015. The Global Impact of Dementia. An Analysis of Prevalence, Incidence, Cost and Trends [Internet]. 2015. Available from: https://www.alzint.org/u/worldalzheimerreport2015summary.pdf

[6] Gorelick PB, Scuteri A, Black SE, DeCarli C, Greenberg SM, Iadecola C, et al. Vascular contributions to cognitive impairment and dementia: A statement for healthcare professionals from the American Heart Association/American Stroke Association. Stroke. 2011;**42**(9): 2672-2713

[7] Blessed G, Tomlinson BE, Roth M. The association between quantitative measures of dementia and of senile change in the cerebral grey matter of elderly subjects. The British Journal of Psychiatry. 1968;**114**(512):797-811

[8] Grinberg LT. Vascular dementia: Current concepts and nomenclature

harmonization. Dementia & Neuropsychologia. 2012;**6**(3):122-126

[9] Assuncao N, Sudo FK, Drummond C, de Felice FG, Mattos P. Metabolic syndrome and cognitive decline in the elderly: A systematic review. PLoS ONE. 2018;**13**(3):e0194990

[10] Yaffe K. The metabolic syndrome, inflammation, and risk of cognitive decline. Journal of the American Medical Association. 2004;**292**(18): 2237

[11] Farina MP, Zhang YS, Kim JK, Hayward MD, Crimmins EM. Trends in dementia prevalence, incidence, and mortality in the United States (2000-2016). Journal of Aging and Health. 2021;**7**:089826432110297

[12] Wolters FJ, Chibnik LB, Waziry R, Anderson R, Berr C, Beiser A, et al. Twenty-seven-year time trends in dementia incidence in Europe and the United States: The Alzheimer Cohorts Consortium. Neurology. 2020;**95**(5): e519-e531

[13] Ozbabalk D, Arslanta D, Tuncer N. The epidemiology of vascular dementia. In: Atwood C, editor. Geriatrics [Internet]. Rijeka: InTechOpen; 2012. Available from: http://www.intechopen.com/books/geriatrics/the-epidemiyology-of-vascular-dementia

[14] Meyer JS, Xu G, Thornby J, Chowdhury MH, Quach M. Is mild cognitive impairment prodromal for vascular dementia like Alzheimer's disease? Stroke. 2002;**33**(8):1981-1985

[15] Ishii H, Meguro K, Yamaguchi S, Ishikawa H, Yamadori A. Prevalence and cognitive performances of vascular cognitive impairment no dementia in Japan: The Osaki?Tajiri Project. European Journal of Neurology. 2007;**14**(6):609-616

[16] Jellinger KA, Attems J. Prevalence and pathology of vascular dementia in the oldest-old. JAD. 2010;**21**(4): 1283-1293

[17] Jellinger K. Current pathogenetic concepts of vascular cognitive impairment. Journal of Neurology, Neurological Science and Disorders. 2016;**2**(1):010-016

[18] Ikejima C, Yasuno F, Mizukami K, Sasaki M, Tanimukai S, Asada T. Prevalence and causes of early-onset dementia in Japan: A population-based study. Stroke. 2009;**40**(8):2709-2714

[19] Garre-Olmo J, Genís Batlle D, del Mar FM, Marquez Daniel F, de Eugenio HR, Casadevall T, et al. Incidence and subtypes of early-onset dementia in a geographically defined general population. Neurology. 2010;**75**(14):1249-1255

[20] Meguro K, Ishii H, Kasuya M, Akanuma K, Meguro M, Kasai M, et al. Incidence of dementia and associated risk factors in Japan: The Osaki-Tajiri Project. Journal of the Neurological Sciences [Internet]. 2007;**260**(1-2): 175-182. Available from: https:// linkinghub.elsevier.com/retrieve/pii/ S0022510X0700319X

[21] Sekita A, Ninomiya T, Tanizaki Y, Doi Y, Hata J, Yonemoto K, et al. Trends in prevalence of Alzheimer's disease and vascular dementia in a Japanese community: The Hisayama Study: Trend in prevalence of dementia in Japan. Acta Psychiatrica Scandinavica. 2010;**122**(4): 319-325

[22] Herrera E, Caramelli P, Silveira ASB, Nitrini R. Epidemiologic survey of dementia in a community-dwelling Brazilian population. Alzheimer Disease and Associated Disorders. 2002;**16**(2): 103-108

[23] Fagundes SD, Silva MT, Thees MFRS, Pereira MG. Prevalence

of dementia among elderly Brazilians: A systematic review. São Paulo Medical Journal. 2011;**129**(1):46-50

[24] CMC B, Azevedo D Jr, Tatsch M, Hototian SR, Moscoso MA, Folquitto J, et al. Estimate of dementia prevalence in a community sample from São Paulo, Brazil. Dementia and Geriatric Cognitive Disorders [Internet]. 2008;**26**(4):291-299. Available from: https://www.karger.com/Article/ FullText/161053

[25] Jia J, Wang F, Wei C, Zhou A, Jia X, Li F, et al. The prevalence of dementia in urban and rural areas of China. Alzheimer's and Dementia [Internet]. 2014;**10**(1):1-9. Available from: https:// onlinelibrary.wiley.com/doi/10.1016/j. jalz.2013.01.012

[26] Hébert R, Lindsay J, Verreault R, Rockwood K, Hill G, Dubois M-F. Vascular dementia: Incidence and risk factors in the Canadian study of health and aging. Stroke. 2000;**31**(7): 1487-1493

[27] Knopman DS, Parisi JE, Boeve BF, Cha RH, Apaydin H, Salviati A, et al. Vascular dementia in a population-based autopsy study. Archives of Neurology. 2003;**60**(4):569-575

[28] Tabet N, Quinn R, Klugman A. Prevalence and cognitive impact of cerebrovascular findings in Alzheimer's disease: A retrospective, naturalistic study. International Journal of Clinical Practice. 2009;**63**(2):338-345

[29] Rockwood K, Wentzel C, Hachinski V, Hogan DB, MacKnight C, McDowell I. Prevalence and outcomes of vascular cognitive impairment. Neurology. 2000;**54**(2):447-447

[30] Fitzpatrick AL, Kuller LH, Ives DG, Lopez OL, Jagust W, Breitner JCS, et al. Incidence and prevalence of dementia in the cardiovascular health study: Incidence of dementia in CHS. Journal

of the American Geriatrics Society. 2004;**52**(2):195-204

[31] Bowler JV. The concept of vascular cognitive impairment. Journal of the Neurological Sciences. 2002;**203-204**: 11-15

[32] Gauthier S, Rockwood K. Does vascular MCI progress at a different rate than does amnestic MCI? International Psychogeriatrics. 2003;**15**(S1):257-259

[33] Engelhardt E, Tocquer C, André C, Moreira DM, Okamoto IH, Cavalcanti JL d S. Vascular dementia: Diagnostic criteria and supplementary exams: Recommendations of the Scientific Department of Cognitive Neurology and Aging of the Brazilian Academy of Neurology. Part I. Dementia & Neuropsychologia. 2011;**5**(4):251-263

[34] Petersen RC. Mild cognitive impairment as a diagnostic entity. Journal of Internal Medicine. 2004;**256**(3): 83-194

[35] Zhao Q, Zhou Y, Wang Y, Dong K, Wang Y. A new diagnostic algorithm for vascular cognitive impairment: The proposed criteria and evaluation of its reliability and validity. Chinese Medical Journal. 2010;**123**(3):311-319

[36] American Psychiatric Association. Diagnostic and Statistical Manual of Mental Disorders. 5th ed. Arlington, VA: American Psychiatric Publishing; 2013. Available from: https://doi.org/10.1176/ appi.books.9780890425596.dsm05

[37] Roman GC, Tatemichi TK, Erkinjuntti T, Cummings JL, Masdeu JC, Garcia JH, et al. Vascular dementia: Diagnostic criteria for research studies: Report of the NINDS-AIREN International Workshop. Neurology. 1993;**43**(2):250-250

[38] Organização Mundial de Saúde. Classificação Estatística Internacional de Doenças e Problemas Relacionados à Saúde - 10a edição (CID-10). 10th ed. São Paulo: Universidade de São Paulo; 1997

[39] Skrobot OA, Black SE, Chen C, DeCarli C, Erkinjuntti T, Ford GA, et al. Progress toward standardized diagnosis of vascular cognitive impairment: Guidelines from the Vascular Impairment of Cognition Classification Consensus Study. Alzheimer's & Dementia. 2018;**14**(3):280-292

[40] Román GC, Sachdev P, Royall DR, Bullock RA, Orgogozo J-M, López-Pousa S, et al. Vascular cognitive disorder: A new diagnostic category updating vascular cognitive impairment and vascular dementia. Journal of the Neurological Sciences. 2004;**226**(1-2): 81-87

[41] Inzitari D, Pracucci G, Poggesi A, Carlucci G, Barkhof F, Chabriat H, et al. Changes in white matter as determinant of global functional decline in older independent outpatients: Three year follow-up of LADIS (leukoaraiosis and disability) study cohort. BMJ. 2009;**339**(1):b2477-b2477

[42] Engelhardt E, Moreira DM, Alves GS, Lanna MEO, Alves CE d O, Ericeira-Valente L, et al. Binswanger's disease and quantitative fractional anisotropy. Arquivos de Neuro-Psiquiatria. 2009;**67**(2a):179-184

[43] Garcia JH, Brown GG. Vascular dementia: Neuropathologic alterations and metabolic brain changes. Journal of the Neurological Sciences. 1992;**109**(2): 121-131

[44] Takeda S, Rakugi H, Morishita R. Roles of vascular risk factors in the pathogenesis of dementia. Hypertension Research [Internet]. 2020;**43**(3):162-167. Available from: http://www.nature. com/articles/s41440-019-0357-9

[45] Erkinjuntti T, Román G, Gauthier S, Feldman H, Rockwood K. Emerging

therapies for vascular dementia and vascular cognitive impairment. Stroke [Internet]. 2004;**35**(4):1010-1017. Available from: https://www.ahajournals.org/doi/10.1161/01.STR.0000120731.88236.33

[46] Gustafson D, Skoog I. Control of vascular risk factors. In: Wahlund L-O, Erkinjuntti T, Gauthier S, editors. Vascular Cognitive Impairment in Clinical Practice [Internet]. Cambridge: Cambridge University Press; 2009. pp. 220-234. Available from: https://www.cambridge.org/core/product/identifier/9780511575976%23c87537-18-1/type/book_part

[47] van der Flier WM, Skoog I, Schneider JA, Pantoni L, Mok V, Chen CLH, et al. Vascular cognitive impairment. Nature Reviews Disease Primers [Internet]. 2018;**4**(1):18003. Available from: http://www.nature.com/articles/nrdp20183

[48] Caramelli P, Barbosa MT. Como diagnosticar as quatro causas mais freqüentes de demência? Revista Brasileira de Psiquiatria. 2002; **24**(suppl 1):7-10

[49] Malloy-Diniz L, Fuentes D, Mattos P. Avaliação Neuropsicológica. 2nd ed. Porto Alegre: Artmed; 2018

[50] Hachinski V, Iadecola C, Petersen RC, Breteler MM, Nyenhuis DL, Black SE, et al. National Institute of Neurological Disorders and Stroke–Canadian Stroke Network Vascular Cognitive Impairment Harmonization Standards. Stroke. 2006;**37**(9):2220-2241

[51] National Institute of Health and Care Excellence. Dementia: Assessment, Management and Support for People Living with Dementia and their Carers [Internet]. 2018. Available from: https://www.nice.org.uk/guidance/ng97/chapter/Recommendations#pharmacological-interventions-for-dementia

[52] Sachdev P, Kalaria R, O'Brien J, Skoog I, Alladi S, Black SE, et al. Diagnostic criteria for vascular cognitive disorders: A VASCOG statement. Alzheimer Disease and Associated Disorders. 2014;**28**(3):206-218

[53] Wardlaw JM, Smith EE, Biessels GJ, Cordonnier C, Fazekas F, Frayne R, et al. Neuroimaging standards for research into small vessel disease and its contribution to ageing and neurodegeneration. The Lancet Neurology. 2013;**12**(8):822-838

[54] Alves GS, O'Dwyer L, Jurcoane A, Oertel-Knöchel V, Knöchel C, Prvulovic D, et al. Different patterns of white matter degeneration using multiple diffusion indices and volumetric data in mild cognitive impairment and Alzheimer patients. PLoS ONE. 2012;**7**(12):e52859

[55] Burgmans S, van Boxtel MPJ, Gronenschild EHBM, Vuurman EFPM, Hofman P, Uylings HBM, et al. Multiple indicators of age-related differences in cerebral white matter and the modifying effects of hypertension. NeuroImage. 2010;**49**(3):2083-2093

[56] Alexopoulos GS, Meyers BS, Young RC, Campbell S, Silbersweig D, Charlson M. 'Vascular depression' hypothesis. Archives of General Psychiatry [Internet]. 1997;**54**(10): 915-22. DOI: 10.1001/archpsyc.1997.01830220033006

[57] Ballard C, Neill D, O'Brien J, McKeith IG, Ince P, Perry R. Anxiety, depression and psychosis in vascular dementia: Prevalence and associations. Journal of Affective Disorders [Internet] 2000;**59**(2):97-106. Available from: https://linkinghub.elsevier.com/retrieve/pii/S0165032799000579

[58] Cummings JL. Frontal-subcortical circuits and human behavior. Journal of Psychosomatic Research 1998;**44**(6):627-628

[59] Gauthier S, Erkinjuntti T. Treatment of cognitive changes. In: Wahlund L-O, Erkinjuntti T, Gauthier S, editors. Vascular Cognitive Impairment in Clinical Practice [Internet]. Cambridge: Cambridge University Press; 2009. pp. 195-199. Available from: https://www.cambridge.org/core/product/identifier/9780511575976%23c87537-15-1/type/book_part

[60] Perng C-H, Chang Y-C, Tzang R-F. The treatment of cognitive dysfunction in dementia: A multiple treatments meta-analysis. Psychopharmacology [Internet]. 2018;**235**(5):1571-1580. Available from: http://link.springer.com/10.1007/s00213-018-4867-y

[61] World Health Organization. Risk Reduction of Cognitive Decline and Dementia. WHO Guidelines [Internet]. 2019. Available from: https://www.who.int/mental_health/neurology/dementia/guidelines_risk_reduction/en/

[62] Brucki SMD, Ferraz AC, de Freitas GR, Massaro AR, Radanovic M, Schultz RR. Treatment of vascular dementia Recommendations of the Scientific Department of Cognitive Neurology and Aging of the Brazilian Academy of Neurology. Dementia & Neuropsychologia. 2011;**5**(4):275-287

[63] Abrisqueta-Gomez J, Canali F, Vieira VLD, Aguiar ACP, Ponce CSC, Brucki SM, et al. A longitudial study of a neuropsychological rehabilitation program in Alzheimer's disease. Arquivos de Neuro-Psiquiatria. 2004;**62**(3b):778-783

Chapter 6

Cerebral Vasospasm: Mechanisms, Pathomorphology, Diagnostics, Treatment

Irina Alexandrovna Savvina,

Yulia Mikhailovna Zabrodskaya, Anna Olegovna Petrova
and Konstantin Alexandrovich Samochernykh

Abstract

Cerebral vessels constriction is one of the leading causes of mortality and disability in patients with acute cerebral circulatory disorders. The most dangerous type of acute cerebrovascular disease accompanied by high mortality is ruptured cerebral aneurysms with subarachnoidal hemorrhage (SAH). Following a constriction of the cerebral vessels on the background of SAH is the reason for brain ischemia. This chapter will focus on the mechanisms of formation of cerebral vascular spasm, pathomorphological aspects of the cerebral vessels constriction, and the stages of vascular spasm—the development of constrictive-stenotic arteriopathy, contractural degeneration of smooth muscle cells, and endothelial damage. We will cover classifications of cerebral vessels constriction by prevalence and severity, modern methods of clinical and instrumental diagnostics and treatment including paroxysmal sympathetic hyperactivity syndrome associated with the development of secondary complications, a longer stay of the patients in the ICU, higher disability and mortality.

Keywords: cerebral vessels constriction, SAH, arteriopathy, cerebral angiography, transcranial Dopplerography, paroxysmal sympathetic hyperactivity syndrome

1. Introduction

This chapter focuses on the problem of cerebral vessels spasm as the reason for brain ischemia. Vessel spastic constriction is one of the leading causes of mortality and disability in patients with ruptured cerebral aneurysms as the most dangerous type of acute cerebral circulatory disorders accompanied by high mortality. In this chapter, we describe the mechanisms of formation of cerebral vessels constriction, including on the background of subarachnoidal hemorrhage and various pathological conditions—migraine, traumatic brain injury, ischemia or hypoxia, and arterial hypertension. Pathomorphological picture of cerebral vessels constriction is described here, smooth muscle role in the constriction of cerebral blood vessels, stages of cerebral blood vessels spasm, the development of constrictive-stenotic arteriopathy, endothelial damage. Diagnostics of cerebral vessels constriction include neurological assessment and data of cerebral angiography, transcranial Dopplerography with quantitative assessment of blood flow. Here is described the classification of cerebral vasospasm by prevalence and severity and its treatment including paroxysmal sympathetic hyperactivity syndrome, neurovegetative stabilization method, and therapeutic hypothermia.

1.1 Determination of cerebral vasospasm

Cerebral vasospasm is understood as a local or diffuse persistent spastic constriction of the smooth muscle elements of the vascular wall of the cerebral arteries, which is accompanied by a decrease in their lumen, that leads to a decrease in blood supply to the brain [1].

1.2 Background of the vasospastic theory of cerebral ischemia

The role of cerebral vasospasm in the genesis of cerebral ischemic disorders is currently the subject of discussion. At the end of the nineteenth century and in the first half of the twentieth century, cerebral vasospasm was considered as one of the leading causes of the development of ischemic stroke. As the methods of in vivo diagnosis of cerebrovascular pathology improved, the vasospastic theory gradually lost its significance. In addition, it was found that the cerebral arteries are one of the least reactive in the body [2]. It is assumed that only under strictly defined conditions, cerebral vasospasm can be the cause of cerebral ischemia, namely, in subarachnoid hemorrhage and, probably, in migraines [1, 3, 4]. At the same time, cerebral vasospasm has recently been considered again as a possible cause of the development of cerebral ischemic disorders during endovascular neurosurgical interventions [5].

2. The mechanisms of formation of cerebral vessels constriction

Until now, it is not completely clear what is the result of cerebral vascular spasm—an increase in the sensitivity of vascular smooth muscle cells to vasoconstrictor effects, an increase in the content of vasoconstrictors in the blood, a violation of the processes of postconstrictor relaxation of blood vessels, or morphological changes in the walls of blood vessels. The cause of vascular spasm can be the direct effect of oxyhemoglobin on the vascular wall, the breakdown products of red blood cells, endothelin, and many other factors [6]. The action of oxyhemoglobin may include direct vasoconstriction, the release of arachidonic metabolites and endothelin from the arterial wall, inhibition of endothelium-dependent vasodilation by removing nitric oxide, damage to perivascular nerves, and stimulation of free radical reactions [7].

2.1 Subarachnoidal hemorrhage and cerebral vessels constriction

Based on the results of the numerous studies, Towart R. identified three groups of factors that affect vascular tone in SAH [8]:

Group 1—Substances that cause vascular spasm (serotonin and its metabolites, catecholamines, histamine, angiotensin, vasopressin, prostaglandins, in particular, prostaglandin F2a, thromboxane A2);

Group 2—Substances that can contribute to the development of arterial spasm (red blood cell breakdown products, thrombin, fibrinogen breakdown products, prostaglandins, histamine, serotonin, and potassium);

Group 3—Factors that increase spasm due to increased sensitivity of vascular constrictors due to activation of the sympathetic nervous system (increased potassium content in the cerebrospinal fluid, the presence of blood components in the cerebrospinal fluid, fibrinogen breakdown products, angiotensin, platelet growth factor, endothelin).

It is known that when the endothelium is damaged against the background of SAH, activation of phospholipid peroxidation of the plasma membrane of a smooth muscle cell occurs, which leads to the accumulation of diacylglycerol, activation of protein kinase C, and prolonged constriction of the vessel wall [9–11]. On the other hand, it is suggested that reactive oxygen species are involved in the activation of protein tyrosine kinase and mitogen-activating protein kinase [12–14]. Against this background, various biological processes are induced—cell proliferation and migration, apoptosis.

Arterial vessels in the area of hemorrhage (directly in the hematoma or washed with bloody liquor) are exposed to biologically active compounds aggressive to the vascular wall—products of blood breakdown and inflammatory reactions [6].

Sympathetic activation after SAH can stimulate inflammatory reactions [7, 15].

Spasm of the cerebral vessels on the background of SAH exists for quite a long time (up to several weeks). It is obvious that the pathophysiological mechanisms of spasms in large cerebral arteries do not exhaust the problems of brain ischemia. Over time, there are ultrastructural changes in the large vessels of the brain (intima compaction, destruction of the endothelium), which leads to its chronic ischemia [4, 5].

Many vasoconstrictor substances (catecholamines, serotonin, prostaglandins, thromboxane A2, hemoglobin, and products of destruction of red blood cells) cause vasospasm through various mechanisms, but the common thing is that they increase the intracellular concentration of free calcium. These processes are controlled by cAMP and cGMP. Therefore, one of the ways to prevent vasospasm is to increase the concentration of cAMP and cGMP, which increase the calcium uptake by the sarcoplasmic reticulum, which, theoretically, should lead to vascular relaxation.

Thus, the pathophysiological mechanisms that lead to cerebral vasoconstriction are complex.

2.2 Mechanisms of formation of cerebral vessels spasm in various pathological conditions

Figure 1 shows the mechanisms of formation of cerebral vascular spasm in various pathological conditions (migraine, traumatic brain injury, ischemia or hypoxia, SAH, arterial hypertension) [2].

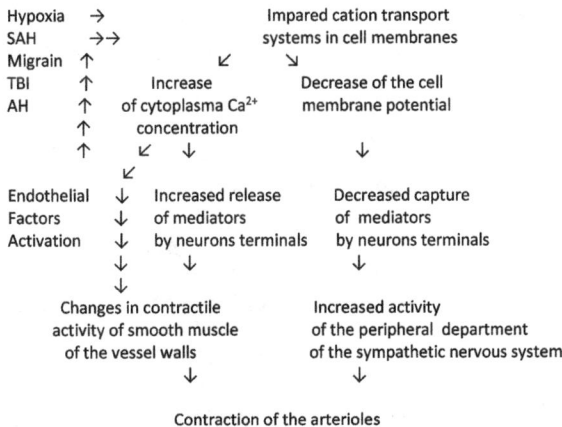

Figure 1.
Formation of cerebral vascular spasm [2].

3. Pathomorphology of cerebral vessels constriction

3.1 Smooth muscle role in the constriction of cerebral blood vessels

Smooth muscle in the cerebral blood vessels is involuntary. It is considered that normally the muscular apparatus of the arteries remains partially reduced and this "basal tone" ensures the maintenance of the necessary level of blood pressure. Increased tone (and pressure) is a result of constriction of the smooth muscle apparatus and narrowing of the artery lumen. Electron microscopic studies have established that three varieties of filaments are involved in the constriction of smooth muscle cells—thin (7 nm), thick (17 nm), and intermediate (continuous). The latter play a leading role in the constriction. They form a continuous system, a kind of network, inside each cell.

There are also so-called dense corpuscles, which act as reference points during the act of constriction. These formations contain a protein (α-actin), which allows us to consider them analogs of Z-plates of striated musculature. The reduction of intermediate filaments leads to the dislocation of thin (actin) and thick (myosin) filaments, their sliding along with each other leads to cell deformation. In the intervals between dense parts, the cytoplasmic membrane bulges outwards. A shrunken cell in a scanning microscope has a "bumpy" surface [16].

3.2 Stages of cerebral blood vessels spasm

Like any pathological process, vasospasm passes through three stages in its development—normal vessel tone → spasm (reversible constriction of the vessel lumen) → irreversible spasm.

The irreversible phase of the pathological spasm is accompanied by damage to the structural elements of the artery wall with the development of contractural degeneration of myocytes, subsequent cell death, and endotheliosis.

Developing arteriopathy is the result of a spasm (constriction) and is manifested by a hemodynamically significant narrowing (stenosis) of the lumen due to intussusceptions (indentation) of the intima and internal parts of the t. media and edema into it [17].

The development of constrictive stenotic arteriopathy against the background of prolonged or chronic vasospasm can be divided into two phases:

- functional spasm and stenosing spasm (contracture).

3.2.1 Arterial spasm (reversible functional state)

Morphological manifestations of spasm of the arteries of the base of the brain (**Figure 2**):

- narrowing of the vessel lumen;

- thickening of the artery wall with the formation of protrusions into the lumen;

- wavy ("corrugated") the stroke of the internal elastic membrane (data);

- change of the horizontal (planar) orientation of the endothelium to the vertical;

- shortening and thickening of myocytes;

- stellate configuration of the myocyte nucleus;

- the wavy course of collagen fibers in adventitia [17–22].

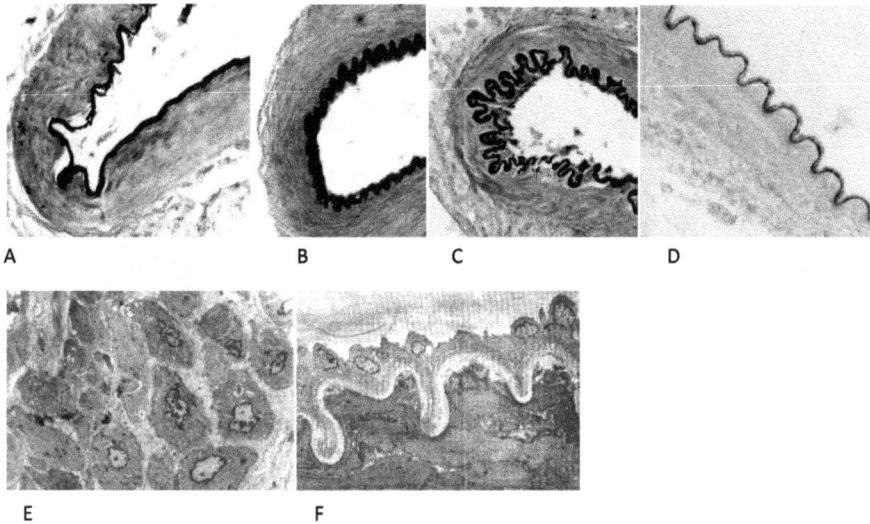

Figure 2.
Morphology of different arterial tones and spasms. A. Atonic state of the artery. Straightened internal elastic membrane, segmentally weakly pronounced folds on the inner surface of the artery. Coloring with orsein on elastic. Magnification 200. B. Increased arterial tone. A corrugated internal elastic membrane without the formation of muscle folds. Coloring with orsein on elastic. Magnification 200. C. Mild spasm. Small folds of the internal elastic membrane with muscle invaginations. Coloring with orsein on elastic. Magnification of 200. D. Moderate spasm. Uniform internal folds of the artery. The color is toluidine blue. Magnification 200. E. Stellate configuration of myocytes and nuclei, the appearance of electron-dense particles in the cytoplasm during constriction. Electronogram.Magnification 200. F. On the surface of the folds of the intima of the spastic artery, the" bulging "endothelium is rounded on the surface and compressed in the depth of the folds. Electronogram.Magnification 750.

3.2.2 Stenosing spasm (contracture)

With prolonged spasm, the following changes in the artery wall are added to the above-listed manifestations of ordinary spasm, leading to additional narrowing of the lumen:

- the formation of large longitudinal folds of the intima, formed due to a sharp reduction in the internal bundles of smooth muscle cells and significantly protruding into the lumen of the vessel;

- hyperhydration of the walls with the accumulation of edematous fluid under the IEM on the tops of the intima folds and aggravation of lumen stenosis. The formation of large folds carries the effect of stenosis—an additional volume appears in the maximally narrowed lumen of the artery, due to which not only the internal relief of the vessel changes but even more its throughput for blood decreases, which is recorded by radiopaque methods of examination and is designated as a vascular spasm (**Figure 3**).

3.2.3 Contractural degeneration (destruction) of smooth muscle cells

A material substrate of irreversible changes in smooth muscle cells with spasm, which are the final of a long stay of the vessel (arteries) in an aggressive environment, contractural degeneration appeared—a variant of irreversible dystrophy, which was not previously listed in the list of such processes in relation to smooth muscle cells. Irreversible damage to the cell myofibrils with the subsequent development of dystrophic changes, colliquation and coagulation necrosis of the nuclei and cytoplasm of the

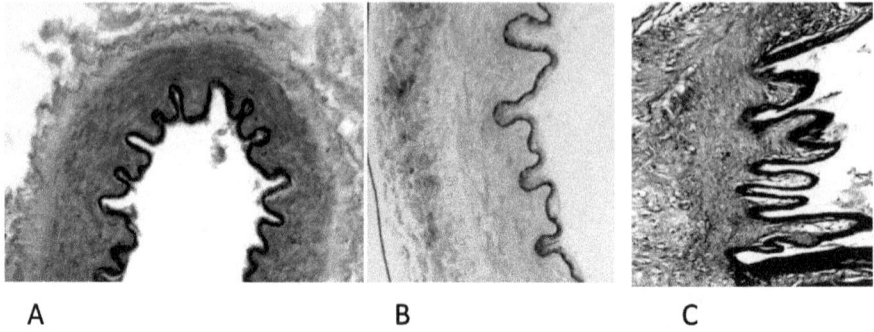

Figure 3.
Constrictive-stenotic arteriopathy ("vasospasm"). A. Deep muscle invaginates forming deep folds stenosing the lumen of the artery. Coloring with orsein on elastic. Increase 200. B. Double-humped invaginates of the muscular membrane, rough deep folds. The color is toluidine blue. Magnification 200. C. There is an accumulation of edematous fluid in the invaginate zone under the internal elastic membrane. Staining with thionine. Magnification of 200.

cell elements of the middle shell, is the result of mechanical rupture of the cell myofibrils with prolonged spasm, developing at 2–4 weeks under the influence of biologically aggressive substances of the spilled blood. The morphogenesis of contractural degeneration, as a special case of myocyte damage, is demonstrated in **Figure 4** [23].

Stages of destructive changes in the contractile apparatus of smooth muscle cells of the arteries of the base of the human brain in constrictive-stenotic arteriopathy [24].

At the top, the smooth muscle cell is in a relaxed state (nucleus, contractile myofibrils: thin, thick, intermediate);

1. A contracted smooth muscle cell. The shape of the cell and the nucleus are changed, actin and myosin contractile fibrils have come into contact (in accordance with the principle of "sliding mechanism");

2. Prolonged spasm (contracture). Destruction of myofilaments;

3. Impregnation of the dead cell with plasma and tissue fluid;

4. Forming layered corpuscles in the dead smooth muscle cells;

5. Formed layered corpuscles;

6. The remains of a cell in the interstitial tissue (**Figure 5**).

3.2.4 Endotheliosis and desquamation of the endothelium

Against the background of prolonged spasm, dystrophic changes in the endothelium are recorded with vacuolization of the cytoplasm and a violation of the connection of endotheliocytes with the basement membrane. The endothelium is "squeezed" into the lumen from the depth of the folds formed during a stenotic spasm. Changes in the endothelium during a spasm and the development of constrictive-stenotic arteriopathy (**Figure 6**):

• endothelial damage (endotheliosis);

• desquamation of the endothelium;

• formation of surface erosions of the intima.

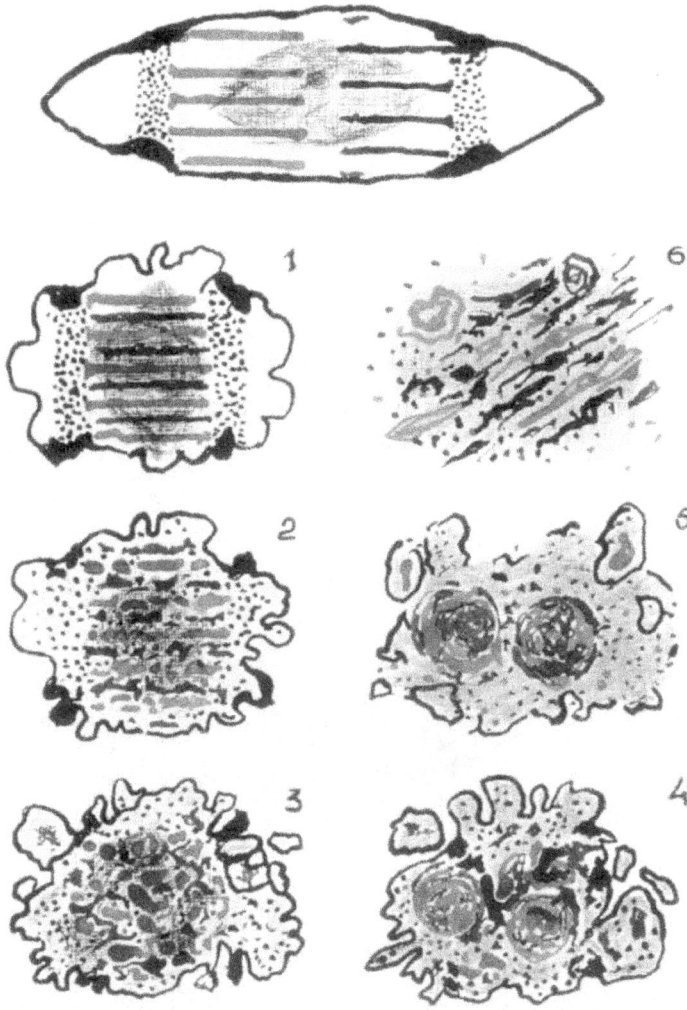

Figure 4.
Damage to smooth muscle cells during prolonged vasospasm (author's drawing of Professor Medvedev Yu.A., 2001).

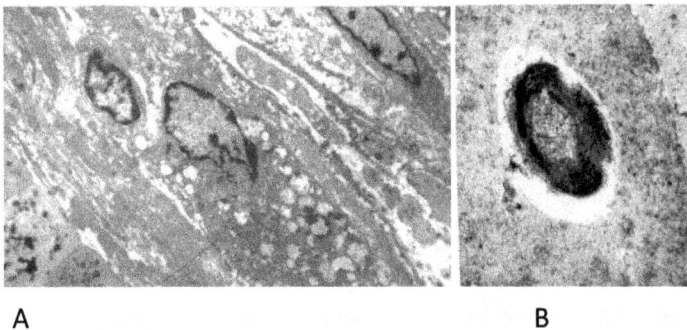

Figure 5.
Damage to smooth muscle cells in contracture degeneration. A. Vacuole dystrophy and myocytolysis. Electronogram.Mag. 2000. B. a layered body made of fragments of fused myofibrils destruction of the functional substrate of the artery wall (smooth muscle it explains the tolerance of blood vessels to drug dilation therapy in constrictive-stenotic arteriopathy Electronogram.Mag. 20000 [24].

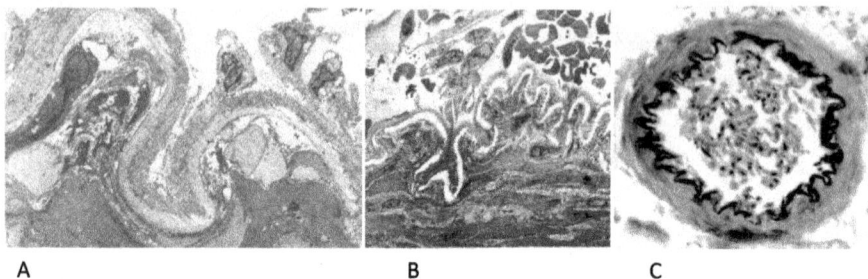

Figure 6.
Constrictive-stenotic arteriopathy ("vasospasm"). Endotheliosis. A. on the surface of the intimate fold, on the right, there is an endothelium with degenerative changes (vacuolized cytoplasm and deformed nucleus), cell decomplexation, and loss of connection with the basement membrane, on the left—the inner surface is devoid of an endothelial layer, in the roughness of the folds there is cellular detritus of a necrotized endotheliocyte, under the inner elastic membrane there is an accumulation of fluid and dystrophically altered myocytes. Electronogram.mag. 2000. B. Desquamation of the endothelium in the zone of pronounced folding of the wall with the erosion of the inner circumference of the artery. There is a desquamated endothelium in the lumen of the spasmed artery. Electronogram.mag. 750. C. Cellular embolus of desquamated endothelium in the lumen of a spasmodic small artery. Coloring with orsein on elastic. mag. 200.

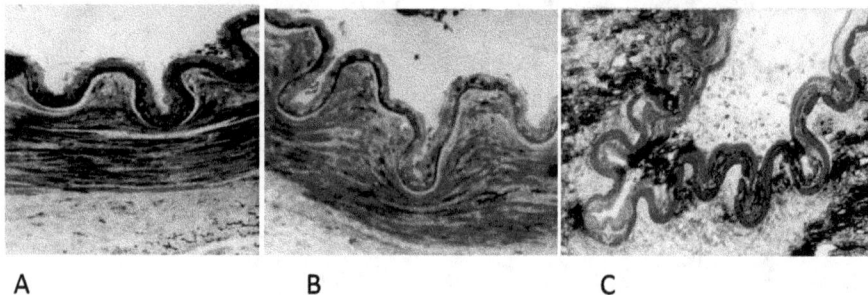

Figure 7.
Stages of constrictive-stenotic arteriopathy. A. Stage of reactive spasm. Reversible phase. B. Stage of stenosing spasm (contracture). C. Stage of edema and destructive changes. The irreversible phase.

Endothelial damage explains the observed endothelial dysfunction. The loss of the endothelium does not yet lead to thrombosis, a violation of the parietal membrane can affect the rheology of the blood.

Thus, vasospasm after intracranial hemorrhages should be considered as a pathological process that develops as a result of prolonged reactive spasm with the development of arteriopathy, consisting in contractural degeneration of myocytes, endotheliosis, and desquamation of the endothelium with the formation of surface erosions (**Figure** 7).

Contractural degeneration occurs not only in aneurismal hemorrhages. It occurs in all those situations when it comes to hemorrhages in the substance of the brain and its membranes. This is a wide range of diseases, including, first of all, hypertension, as well as other diseases accompanied by arterial hypertension (kidney diseases, endocrinopathy, hemorrhagic diathesis of various nature, traumatic brain injury, surgical brain injury, etc.) [4].

4. Diagnostics of cerebral vessels constriction

4.1 Neurological assessment

Neurological examination is the main clinical tool for the diagnosis of stroke and cerebral vasospasm in particular. The diagnosis of symptomatic vasospasm is based on the appearance of focal or global neurological deterioration. Fluctuation of the level of consciousness, negative dynamics in the form of an increase in the focal neurological deficit, and deprivation of the level of consciousness to stun, sopor up to coma require immediate CT scan of the brain with cerebral angiography. In patients with verified SAH, the condition at admission is assessed on the Hunt-Hess scale [25]. The state at discharge—according to the Glasgow outcome scale [26].

The stimulation of the higher cortical center of the sympathetic nervous system — the insular cortex—with blood spilled due to SAH is realized in a sympathetic "storm" or paroxysmal sympathetic hyperactivity syndrome (PSH). PSH is associated with the development of secondary complications, a longer stay of the patient in the ICU, higher disability, and mortality [27, 28].

Timely and adequate prevention and therapy of the syndrome improves the functional result [29, 30]. Criteria for PSH syndrome and differential criteria are present in **Tables 1** and **2**.

Indicators/points	0	1	2	3
Main criteria				
Pulse rate	<100	110–119	120–139	>140
BP syst	<140	140–159	160–179	>180
Breath rate	<18	18–23	24–29	>30
Kerdo index	0	+1 – +10	+10 – +20	>+21
T C	<37	37–37.9	38–38.9	>40
Increased muscle tone (points)	0	1–2	3	4–5
Frequency of episodes of vegetative instability (in 24 h)	No	3	6	>6
Additional criteria				
Level of consciousness (points) (GCS)	15–14	14–13	12–10	<10
Hyperhydros	No	+	++	+++
Skin hyperemia	no	+	++	+++
Albumin g/l	34–48	28–34	22–28	<22
EEG signs of irrigation of diencephalic structures	no	+	++	+++

Interpretation of results:
0—no; 1–7 p according to the main criteria, no more than 5p according to additional criteria—weakly expressed PSH syndrome; 8–14 p according to the main criteria, no more than 10 p according to additional criteria—moderate PSH syndrome; 15–21 p-according to the main criteria, 10–15 p according to additional criteria- pronounced PSH syndrome.

Table 1.
Criteria for PSH syndrome.

Indicators/points	1	2	3
ΔT C	>0.5	>0.7	>1
Procalcitonin test (qualitative method)	>0.5	>2	>10
Pain	+	++	+++
Pulse rate	80–99	60–79	<60
BP syst	90–100	80–90	<80
T	<36	<35.5	<35

Interpretation of the results: 1–5 p—possible combination with other conditions that require additional diagnosis and treatment; 5–11 p—PSH syndrome is doubtful or is not leading; 11–18 p—PSH syndrome is excluded.
Notes: The assessment is carried out only under the condition of normovolemia, pO2 > 60 mmHg or SpO2 > 85%, pCO2 < 50 mmHg, glycemia > 3.5 mmol/L. DT C - the difference between rectal and axial temperatures; Kerdo index = 100× (1-ADdiast/HR); + weak severity of the sign +. ++ moderate severity of the sign ++. +++ strong severity of the sign +++. The level of consciousness is assessed according to the Glasgow Coma Scale. The assessment of muscle tone is made according to the Ashworth spasticity scale.

Table 2.
Differential criteria.

Pain syndrome assessment in patients with preserved consciousness can be performed according to a 5-point verbal pain assessment scale [31], where 1 point = +; 2–3 points = ++; and 4 points = +++.

The assessment of the level of sympathetic hyperactivity is made at least once a day. The use of differential criteria for the initial and each subsequent assessment is mandatory.

4.2 Instrumental diagnostics of cerebral vasospasm

Instrumental diagnosis of vascular diseases of the brain and cerebral vasospasm, in particular, is based on the joint use of methods of radiation and ultrasound diagnostics.

4.2.1 Cerebral angiography

The "gold standard" for the diagnosis of cerebral vasospasm remains cerebral angiography. The angiographic diagnosis of cerebral vasospasm is established by the presence of local or diffuse narrowing of the cerebral arteries (**Figures 8** and **9**).

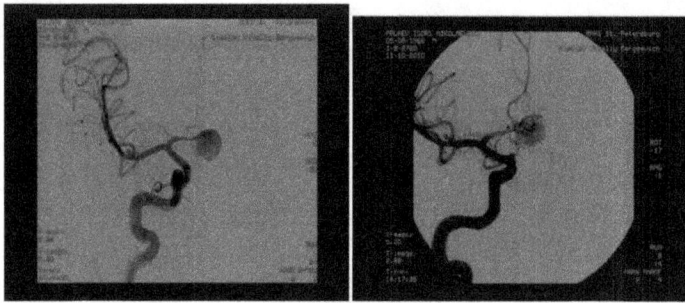

Figure 8.
Cerebral angiography. Multiple cerebral aneurysms: ACA, right MCA in patient P., 45 years old. Cerebral vasospasm detected in the A1 segment right ACA.

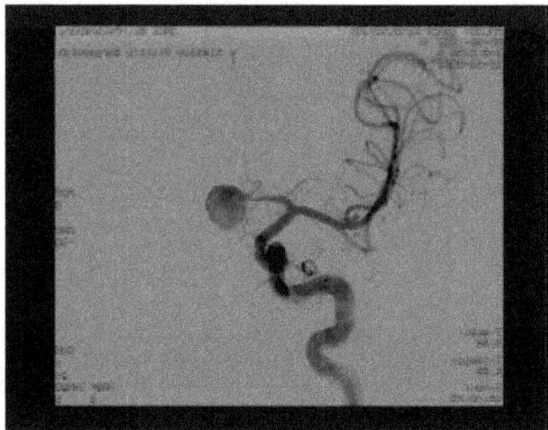

Figure 9.
Local cerebral vasospasm of the A1 segment of the left ACA developed during embolization of the left ACA sac aneurysm (9, 1 × 7, 8 × 6, 1 mm).

4.2.2 Transcranial dopplerography

The possibilities of diagnosing cerebral vasospasm, including its initial stages, have expanded after the introduction of the transcranial Dopplerography method into clinical practice [3].

Ultrasound assessment of blood flow in the cerebral arteries is the most mobile method of screening, dynamic observation, and monitoring of the condition of patients with acute cerebral circulatory insufficiency. In acute cerebral ischemia due to the development of cerebral vasospasm, the prognostic marker and the purpose of monitoring are universal and reproducible characteristics—the flow direction, the type of spectrum, the value of the cerebral blood flow velocity, and the auto-regulatory reserve [3, 32–34].

In cerebral vasospasm, an increase in linear blood flow velocities and, above all, the maximum systolic velocity (or frequency), as well as a violation of cerebro-vascular reactivity, is recorded. Thus, in cerebral vasospasm, the Doppler picture is similar to stenosis and is usually observed in several cerebral arteries [3]. The initial stage of angiospasm is diagnosed when the peak systolic blood flow rate in the middle cerebral artery (MCA) increases to 120 cm/s. With a moderate degree of vasospasm, its value varies from 120 to 200 cm/s, and with severe vasospasm, it exceeds 200 cm/s [34, 35].

With all the variety of pathogenetic variants of damage to the cerebral vascular bed, there are several diagnostically important parameters of the Doppler signal, the changes of which are universal and reproducible, such as the direction of flow relative to the source of ultrasound radiation, the type of spectrum, and the value of the maximum systolic and minimum diastolic velocity [3, 33].

4.2.3 The quantitative assessment of blood flow

The quantitative assessment of blood flow in the arteries of the brain is based both on the directly measured parameters of the Dopplerogram (amplitude, frequency distribution, pulse variations) and on various calculated indices.

The most popular measured Doppler parameter is the flow rate:

- Maximum systolic blood flow velocity (Vsist);

- End diastolic blood flow velocity (Vdiast);

- Average rate per cardiac cycle (MenV);

- Average speed per systole (Vms).

The flow rate is a reference value for arterial vessels with certain characteristics that are close to constant (diameter, depth). Initially, it is assumed that in the absence of structural anomalies and vascular diseases that form the cerebral arterial system, the absolute values of blood flow parameters at rest are constant for a particular person, and their deviations during functional loads (hypoxia, physical exertion, etc.) correspond to the range of the autoregulation reserve.

Based on the indicated parameters characterizing the spectral curves, calculated coefficients have been developed that allow us to quantitatively describe the normal and pathological features of the received signal. The most common methods used for the clinical assessment of blood flow parameters are as follows:

- Circulatory resistance index (RI);

- Pulsatility index (PI);

- Systolic-diastolic index (ISD);

- Spectral Expansion Index (SBI);

- Coefficient of asymmetry (KA);

- Pulse wave rise index (PPI).

Absolute values of blood flow velocity play an important role in assessing the reserve of collateral circulation or calculating the transmission pulsation index (the ratio of velocities in the extra-and intracranial segments of the carotid basin arteries) in cerebral vasospasm.

In addition, all judgments about the quantitative values of the tonic component of the dislocated vessel, the state of the resistive segment of the cerebral arterial pool, and reactive changes during the period of functional stress are also derived from the analysis of the velocity parameters [35].

Turning to the absolute values, it is necessary to take into account some features of the distribution of speed parameters along with the cerebral arteries, due to a combination of physiological and instrumental reasons. These features are manifested by the physiological hierarchy of values of the linear velocity of blood flow in the cerebral and precerebral arteries. At the extracranial level—internal carotid artery > external carotid artery > vertebral artery. At the intracranial level—middle cerebral artery > anterior cerebral artery > internal carotid artery > posterior cerebral artery > main artery > vertebral artery [32].

Between the arteries of the large anastomosis of the base of the brain (Willis circle), the predominance of speed in the middle cerebral artery over the speed in the anterior cerebral artery and posterior cerebral arteries fits into the 20% range [34]. The flow along the main artery is usually always higher than in the best of the vertebral arteries. The normative value of the coefficient of asymmetry between the same carotid arteries of the different sides should not exceed 20%, a 30% difference in speed indicators is permissible for vertebral arteries. Taking into account the anatomical features (the formation of the right arterial sections from the brachiocephalic trunk), lower values are more often recorded in the right vertebral arteries and the internal carotid artery.

Thus, the diagnosis of cerebral vasospasm is based on the data of neurological symptoms, data of cerebral angiography, and the results of transcranial Dopplerography. When comparing instrumental and clinical data, reversible neurological symptoms are usually registered in patients with moderate vessels constriction, and persistent neurological deficit—in severe vasospasm.

5. Classification of cerebral vasospasm

According to transcranial Dopplerography of brain vessels angiospasm is assessed by three degrees of severity: at a blood flow rate of <120 cm/s- I degree, 120–200 cm/s - II degree, >200 cm/s- III degree; by prevalence—vascular spasm of one carotid area-local (segmental), vascular spasm in both carotid areas—widespread (multisegmental), spasm of carotid and vertebrobasilar areas-total (diffuse).

The severity of cerebral vasospasm during endovascular neurosurgery is assessed according to Atkinson P. classification [32].

6. Treatment of cerebral vessels constriction

Treatment of patients with acute disorders of cerebral circulation requires early determination of the causes of acute cerebrovascular accidents, as well as a dynamic assessment of pathogenetic processes.

Previous studies have shown that 13–30% of patients with SAH suffered clinical deterioration due to an ischemic event secondary to cerebral vasospasm, and approximately 50% of these patients either had a long-term pathology or died as a result of such an event [7, 36–39]. Angiographic vasospasm has been reported to occur in 50–70% of patients with SAH [38–40]. A number of researches aimed to identify early predictors of vasospasm after SAH, since such identification could provide more effective prevention of vasospasm and subsequently lead to better neurological outcomes [41].

Vasospasm, which develops in a number of cases during endovascular neurosurgical interventions, is considered a possible cause of perioperative cerebral ischemia [5]. The frequency of subarachnoid hemorrhage (SAH) is 15–18 per 100 thousand people per year [42]. The main causes of death in patients with a ruptured cerebral aneurysm are the direct influence of spilled blood, hydrocephalus and ischemic complications resulting from vasospasm. If the first two causes are coped with more successfully due to the improvement of microsurgical neurosurgical techniques of aneurysm operations and methods of hydrocephalus treatment, then vasospasm and related ischemic complications occupy a leading place among the complications [5, 42].

It was revealed that vasospasm of the I and II degrees is effectively treated conservatively and has no significant effect on the clinical outcome, and diffuse vasospasm of the III degree negatively affects the outcomes and requires the use of endovascular angioplasty and intraarterial pharm angioplasty [43, 44].

It is known that vasospasm appears on the fourth day, increases to 14–17 days, and gradually decreases to 21–30 days.

Figure 10 shows a Dopplerographic picture of cerebral vasospasm of the III degree on the 16th day from the rupture of the ACA aneurysm.

Dopplerography is performed in dynamics in all patients with detected vasospasm in order to determine the effectiveness of treatment. Against the background of positive neurological dynamics, by the end of the fourth week of the disease, most patients have both a general and regional decrease in speed indicators, which is associated with overcoming edema, reducing the volume of brain tissue in the affected pool, restoring the compliance of perfusion capabilities with the metabolic and functional needs of the preserved areas of the brain.

The lengthening of the period of instability of speed parameters or significant fluctuations in absolute values can serve as a marker of an unfavorable prognosis of the deepening of the ischemia process (progredient course), which undoubtedly serves as a basis for clarifying the etiological and/or pathogenetic factor, searching for errors in the choice of therapeutic tactics.

The Fisher CT scale, which evaluates the amount of blood in any cracks or tanks, as well as the presence of intraventricular hemorrhage or intracerebral hemorrhage, is widely used to identify patients with a high risk of developing cerebral vasospasm after SAH [45, 46]. The Fisher CT scale is widely used to identify patients with a high risk of developing cerebral vasospasm after SAH [45, 46]. Vasospasm, according to Fischer's classification, is directly proportional to the outpouring of blood in the basal cisterns (**Figure 11**).

According to this classification, patients with intracerebral hematomas (ICH) and intraventricular hemorrhages (IVH) are at high risk of developing vasospasm [47]. Despite the widespread protocols for the prevention and treatment of vasospasm in recent years, the introduction of endovascular technologies (balloon angioplasty, pharm angioplasty), the results are still unsatisfactory.

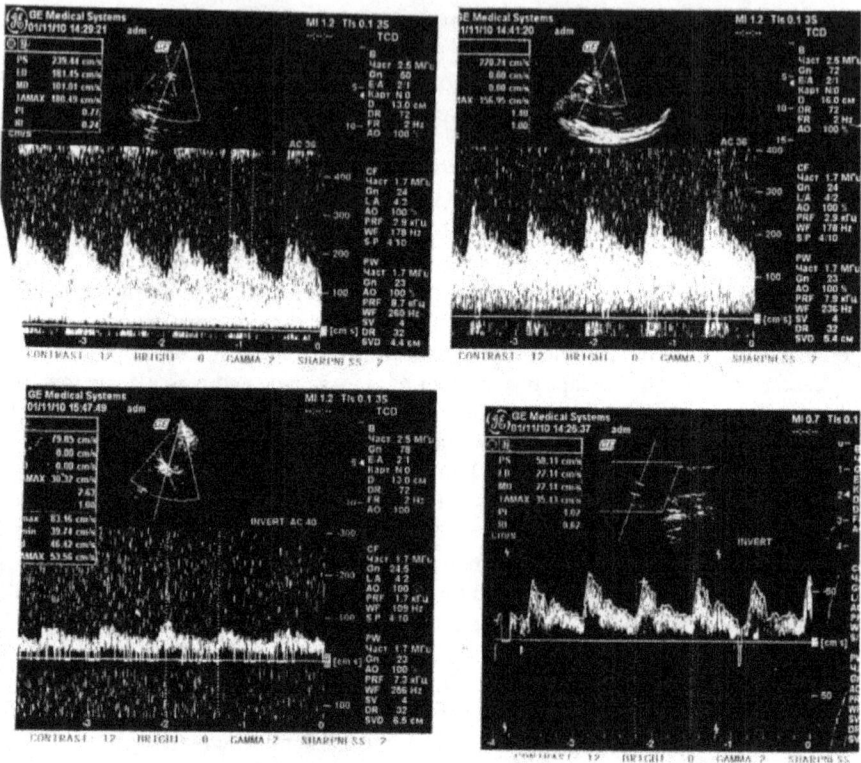

Figure 10.
Cerebral vasospasm of the III st. in both MCA (D < S) in patient M. on the 16th day from a rupture of the ACA aneurysm. Doppler study data.

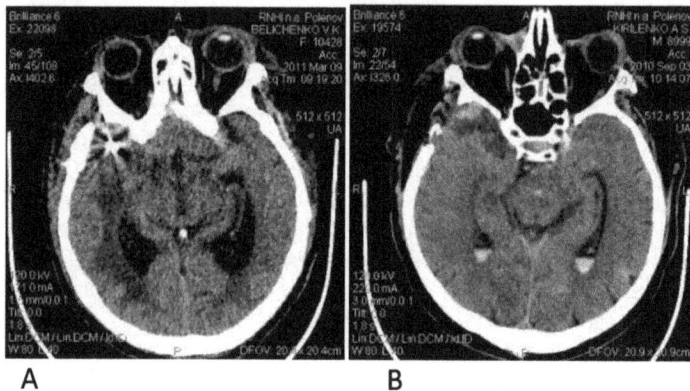

A   B

Figure 11.
Fisher CT III-IY in patients with a cerebral aneurysm, right ACA-ACA (A), left ACA-ACA (B).

Japanese researchers have shown that the amount of blood on computed tomography (CT) is a predictor of cerebral vasospasm after SAH [48]. However, the influence of the location of blood on the frequency of vasospasm remains unclear. The authors retrospectively evaluated the relationship of blood volumes in individual components (tanks and slits) of computed tomography with angiographic vascular spasm after SAH [49–51]. The study included 149 patients with SAH who were scheduled for clipping of a cerebral aneurysm. The amount of subarachnoid blood was classified according to the Fisher CT scale. The amount of subarachnoid blood in five tanks or three slits was also estimated on the SAH scale from 0 to 3 (0 - no blood, 3 - completely filled with blood) [52, 53]. Spasm of the cerebral vessels was diagnosed according to the results of angiography. The researchers obtained the results according to which angiographic vasospasm developed in 51 of 149 patients (34%). Of these, 26 patients had neurological symptoms. The Fisher CT and SAH scores in the right and left Sylvian fissures and suprasellar cisterns were significantly higher in patients with angiographic vasospasm than in patients without it. One-dimensional logistic regression analysis showed that a high level of Fisher CT and high SAH scores in the right and left Sylvian fissure and suprasellar cisterns were predictors of angiographic vasospasm. Multivariate analysis showed that the SAH score in the right Sylvian fissure was an independent predictor of angiographic vasospasm (odds ratio, 3.6; 95% confidence interval (CI), 1.7–7.7; $P = 0.01$) [48].

Activation of the sympathetic nervous system is associated with the development of vasospasm [54–58]. Peerless et al. [54] indicated that vessels removed from direct contact with blood showed reactive narrowing 1 week after SAH, suggesting that cerebral vasospasm may be mediated by a central control mechanism acting through the sympathetic nervous system. Bunc et al. in an experiment on rabbits [55] demonstrated that the influence of the noradrenergic blockade of cerebral noradrenergic areas of the hypothalamus and brain stem prevents vasospasm in circumstances similar to SAH by way of exclusion of the activity of the sympathetic nervous system.

It is well known that the cardiovascular centers of the brain stem are involved in the regulation of cardiac function through sympathetic and parasympathetic efferents [2]. However, recent data have shown that supratentorial centers can also participate in the regulation of the cardiovascular system. Hirashima et al. [59] showed that the amount of SAH in the right Sylvian fissure was independently associated with abnormal ECG changes in patients with SAH, and the degree of the amount of SAH in the right Sylvian fissure was a better predictor of ECG changes than the degree of Fisher CT. These authors suggested that, since the insula cortex is an important site for controlling autonomic function with a right-sided predominance of sympathetic cardiovascular effects, blood in the right Sylvian fissure may stimulate the insula cortex, which leads to sympathetic cardiovascular effects, such as ECG changes. Sympathetic activation can activate inflammatory reactions [7, 15]. Yoshimoto et al. [15] reported that patients with SAC with systemic inflammatory response syndrome had a higher probability of cerebral vasospasm upon admission. Recently, Kato et al. [60] demonstrated that inhibition of sympathetic activation by beta-adrenergic receptor antagonists reduces the levels of proinflammatory cytokines in the cerebrospinal fluid in a rat model of SAH.

Usually, vasospasm is more pronounced on the side of the aneurysm and in the vessels carrying the aneurysm. All patients receive infusion therapy with the calcium channel blocker nimodipine (60 mg every 4 hours). As the degree and prevalence of vasospasm increases, the outcomes worsen, but this does not reach a significant degree, since the cause of fatal and unsatisfactory outcomes in patients with ICH is mainly the volume effect of hematoma, edema, and dislocation of the brain.

Prophylaxis of local cerebral ischemia and cerebral vasospasm following temporary occlusion of the afferent artery during surgical clipping cerebral aneurysm was proposed with short intervals of vessels occlusion in combination with intraoperative intravenous administration of Inosine+Nicotinamide+Riboflavin+Succinic Acid (20,0 ml). Such tactics expands the tolerability to artery occlusion in patients operated in the "cold" period, reduces the possibility of neurological deficit, reduces the recovery period and resuscitation bed-day after neurosurgery [61]. Outcomes in patients with IVH and ICH + IVH were also analyzed depending on the degree and prevalence of vasospasm [1]. According to the data of a number of authors, starting from the second degree of widespread vasospasm, the share of unsatisfactory outcomes and mortality increases sharply [42].

According to the data available in the literature, angiospasm of the I and II degrees did not have a significant effect on the condition and outcome of the disease, but diffuse vasospasm was an independent factor aggravating both the condition and the outcome of the disease [1].

Angiospasm is often observed in patients with ICH and IVH due to the rupture of aneurysms. Taking into account the occurrence and increase of vessels construction, starting from 4 days after hemorrhage, early diagnosis of patients with SAH and hospitalization in specialized vascular neurosurgical centers will allow, along with the shutdown of the aneurysm from the bloodstream, also on the first–fourth day to sanitize the basal cisterns, which largely prevents the occurrence of vasospasm. Conservative treatment with modern drugs is quite effective in patients with angiospasm of I and II degrees. Such an angiospasm has no significant effect on the condition of patients and the outcome of the disease.

Diffuse angiospasm of the III degree is an independent factor that worsens the outcome in patients with aneurysmal ICH and IVH, conservative treatment is ineffective in most cases, therefore, it requires more active treatment in the form of balloon angioplasty and intraarterial pharm angioplasty.

In the diagnosis of cerebral vasospasm of II–III degree and PSH syndrome in patients with SAH, conservative treatment is carried out:

Mild PSH syndrome (1–7 points) - pharmacotherapy—beta-blockers, phenytoin, NSAIDs; physical methods-therapeutic hypothermia.

Moderate PSH syndrome (8–14 points) - pharmacotherapy—beta-blockers, phenytoin, alpha-2 adrenoagonist, NSAIDs; physical methods - therapeutic hypothermia.

Severe PSH syndrome (14–21 points) - neurovegetative stabilization (opioid analgesic, alpha-2 adrenoagonist, hypnotics); physical methods—therapeutic hypothermia (craniocerebral hypothermia).

The duration of therapy is determined individually, after a repeated assessment of the patient's condition.

6.1 Neurovegetative stabilization

Neurovegetative stabilization in the intensive care program for cerebral vasospasm and acute cerebral injury implies the creation of conditions for the absence of debilitating sympathicotonia and the implementation of long-term economical adaptation associated with the predominance of the parasympathetic tone of the autonomic nervous system. It includes intravenous administration of the opioid analgesic fentanyl 0.5–1 mcg/kg/h, alpha-2 adrenoagonists (clonidine 0.2–0.7 mcg/kg/h or dexmedetomidine 0.2–0.5 mcg/kg/h), sodium thiopental 2–4 mg/kg/h [62].

6.2 Therapeutic hypothermia

Apply physical cooling methods to maintain normothermy—craniocerebral hypothermia, which consists in lowering the temperature of the scalp to 5–8°C with the help of helmets cooled by circulating fluid, to maintain the skin temperature at a constant level during the entire cooling session. The cooling duration is from 12 hours to 7 days, with an increase in temperature after the cooling is stopped repeat the procedure, carry out until a stable normothermy is achieved, do not allow the body temperature to drop below 35.5°C; it is permissible to use other cooling methods to maintain normothermy [63].

7. Conclusion

The understanding of the nature of cerebral vessels constriction is not clear thoroughly. To ensure adequate treatment, a rapid diagnostics of cerebral vessels constriction and its nature and cause is necessary. The development of secondary complications, a longer stay of the patients in the ICU, higher disability, and mortality are associated with cerebral vessels constriction. In our opinion, it is necessary to start treatment of cerebral vessels spasm of II–III degree and PSH syndrome in patients with SAH, aneurysmal ICH, and IVH after its verification as soon as possible. Specialized neurosurgical and neurological departments (ICU) allow for modern dynamic neurological and instrumental assessment and specific therapy and surgical intervention.

Acknowledgements

We express our deep gratitude to the teachers—Professors of the Polenov Russian Scientific Research Institute of Neurosurgery—Yuri N. Zubkov, George S. Tigliev, Yuri V. Zotov, Yuri A. Medvedev, Viktor E. Olyushin, Anatoly N. Kondratyev, who influenced our scientific views and clinical experience.

Conflict of interest

There is no conflict of interest.

Abbreviations

AH	arterial hypertention
cAMP	cyclical adenosine-monophosphate
cGMP	cyclical guanosine-monophosphate
CT	computer tomography
ACA	anterior cerebral arteria, anterior communicante arteria
MCA	middle cerebral arteria
SAH	subarachnoidal hemorrhage
TBI	traumatic brain injury
PSH	paroxysmal sympathetic hyperactivity
IVH	intraventricular hemorrhage
ICH	intracerebral hemorrhage
ICU	intensive care unite

Author details

Irina Alexandrovna Savvina*, Yulia Mikhailovna Zabrodskaya,
Anna Olegovna Petrova and Konstantin Alexandrovich Samochernykh
Russian Polenov Scientific Research Neurosurgical Institute—Branch of the
National Almazov Medical Research Centre of Ministry of Health of Russian
Federation, Saint Petersburg, Russian Federation

*Address all correspondence to: irinasavvina@mail.ru

IntechOpen

References

[1] Henneritsi MG, Zh B, Sacco RL. Stroke: Klin. Manual: Translated From English. Moscow: MEDpress-inform; 2008. p. 224

[2] Shuleshova NV, Vishnevsky AA, Kulchitsky VA. The Brain Stem. Clinical and Pathophysiological Correspondences. St. Petersburg: Folio; 2016. p. 356

[3] Kuznetsov AN, Voznyuk IA. Handbook of Cerebral Dopplerography. St. Petersburg: Military Medical Academy; 1997. 100 p

[4] Kuznetsov AN. Modern principles of treatment of multifocal atherosclerosis. Vestn. nats. Medico-Surgical Center. 2008;**3**(1):78-83

[5] Shevchenko YL, Kuznetsov AN, Kucherenko SS, Bolomatov NV, Germanovich VV, Sagildina YO, et al. Cerebral vasospasm during endovascular neurosurgical operations on the cerebral vessels. Bulletin of Pirogov National Medical and Surgical Center. 2010;**5**(4):12-16

[6] Xiao M, Li K, Feng H, Zhang L, Yu C. Neurovascular mechanism of autoregulation of cerebral blood flow after hemorrhagic stroke SAH. Nervous Plasticity. 2017;**2017**:5819514

[7] Kolias AG, Sen J, Belli A. Pathogenesis of cerebral vasospasm following aneurismal subarachnoid hemorrhage: Putative mechanisms and novel approaches. Journal of Neuroscience Research. 2009;**87**(1):1-11

[8] Towart R. The pathophysiology of cerebral vasospasm, and pharmacological approaches to its management. Acta Neurochirurgica (Wien). 1982;**63**(1-4):253-258. DOI: 10.1007/BF01728879

[9] Takuwa Y, Matsui T, Abe Y, Nagafuji T, Yamashita K, Asano T. Alterations in protein kinase C activity and membrane lipid metabolism in cerebral vasospasm after subarachnoid hemorrhage. Journal of Cerebral Blood Flow & Metabolism. 1993;**13**(3):409-415. DOI: 10.1038/jcbfm.1993.55

[10] Matsui T, Asano T. Protein kinase C and vasospasm. Journal of Neurosurgery. 1996;**85**(6):1197-1198. DOI: 10.3171/jns.1996.85.6.1197

[11] Clower BR, Yamamoto Y, Cain L, Haines DE, Smith RR. Endothelial injury following experimental subarachnoid hemorrhage in rats: Effects on brain blood flow. Anatomical Record. 1994;**240**(1):104-114. DOI: 10.1002/ar.1092400110

[12] Davis RJ. The mitogen-activated protein kinase signal transduction pathway. Journal of Biological Chemistry. 1993;**268**(20):14553-14556

[13] Tournier C, Thomas G, Pierre J, Jacquemin C, Pierre M, Saunier B. Mediation by arachidonic acid metabolites of the H_2O_2-induced stimulation of mitogen-activated protein kinases (extracellular-signal-regulated kinase and c-Jun NH2-terminal kinase). European Journal of Biochemistry. 1997;**244**(2):587-595. DOI: 10.1111/j.1432-1033.1997.00587.x

[14] Hossain MI, Marcus JM, Lee JH, Garcia PL, Singh V, Shacka JJ, et al. Restoration of CTSD (cathepsin D) and lysosomal function in stroke is neuroprotective. Autophagy. 2021;**17**(6):1330-1348. DOI: 10.1080/15548627.2020.1761219. Epub 2020 May 25

[15] Yoshimoto Y, Tanaka Y, Hoya K. Acute systemic inflammatory response syndrome in subarachnoid hemorrhage. Stroke. 2001;**32**:1989-1993

[16] Rice RV, Moses JA, McManus GM, et al. The organization of contractile

fibers in the smooth muscles of mammals. Journal of Cell Biology. 1970;**47**:183-196

[17] Medvedev YA, Zubkov YN, Zakaryavichyus ZZ. Poshemorrhagic constrictive-stenotic arteriopathy as an integral part of cerebral vasospasm. Neurosurgery. 1998;**19**(1):22-27

[18] Alksne JF, Greenhut JH. Experimental chronic vasospasm of the brain, including catecholamine. Myonecrosis in the vessel wall. Journal of Neurosurgery. 1974;**417**:440-445

[19] Findlay JM, Weir BKA, et al. Changes in the arterial wall during cerebral vascular spasm. Neurosurgery. 1989;**25**:736-746

[20] Hughes JT, Shianchi PM. Spasm of the cerebral artery. Histological examination in Necropsy of blood vessels in subarachnoid hemorrhage. Journal of Neurosurgery. 1978;**48**:515-525

[21] Iwasa K, Bernanke DH, Smith RR, et al. Non-muscular narrowing of the arteries after subarachnoid hemorrhage: The role of platelet-derived growth factors. Neurosurgery. 1993;**34**:40-45

[22] Meiber MR, Okada T, Bark DH. Morphological changes in the cerebral arteries after subarachnoid hemorrhage. Neurosurgery Clinics of North America. 1990;**1**:417-432

[23] Medvedev YA, Bersnev VP, Nikiforov, Zabrodskaya BM, Y, Zakaryavicius ZZM. Contractural degeneration of smooth muscle cells of the cerebral arteries in the hemorrhage zone after rupture of aneurysms. In: Medvedev YA, editor. Scientific Discoveries in the Russian Neurosurgical Institute of prof. A. L. Polenov. St. Petersburg: "ASTER-X"; 2002. p. 175. ISBN: 5-900356-28-0

[24] Medvedev YA, Zakaryavichus ZZ. Contractural degeneration of smooth muscle cells of the cerebral arteries as the reason of tolerance to pharmacotherapy in posthemorragic period of cerebral aneurysm. Far Eastern Medical Journal. 2002;**3**:134-136. Available from: https://cyberleninka.ru/article/n/kontrakturnaya-degeneratsiya-gladkomyshechnogo-apparata-kak-prichina-tolerantnosti-k-lekarstvennoy-terapii-v-postgemoragicheskom

[25] Hunt W, Hess R. Surgical risk associated with the time of intervention in the treatment of intracranial aneurysms. Journal of Neurosurgeon. 1968;**28**(1):14-20

[26] Jennet B, Bond M. Assessment of the outcome after severe brain damage. The Lancet. 1975;**1**(7905):480-484

[27] Bagley IJ, Nicholls JL, Felmingham KL, Crooks J, Gurka JA, Wade LD. Dysautonomia after a traumatic brain injury: A forgotten syndrome? Journal of Neurology, Neurosurgery, and Psychiatry. 1999;**67**:39-43

[28] Baguli IJ, Heriseanu RE, Gurka JA, Nordenbo A, Cameron ID. Gabapentin in the treatment of dysautonomia after severe traumatic brain injury: A case series. Journal of Neurology, Neurosurgery, and Psychiatry. 2007;**78**:539-541

[29] Compton E. Syndrome of paroxysmal sympathetic hyperactivity after traumatic traumatic brain injury. Nurses Clinics of North America. 2018;**53**(3):459-467. DOI: 10.1016/j.cnur. 2018.05.003

[30] Perks I, Bagley IJ, Knott MT, Menon DK. Review of paroxysmal sympathetic hyperactivity after acquired brain injury. Annals of Neurology. 2010;**68**(2):126-135. DOI: 10.1002/ana.22066

[31] Frank AJM, Moll JMH, Hort JF. A comparison of three ways of measuring

pain. Rheumatology. 1982;**21**(4):211-217.
DOI: 10.1093/rheumatology/21.4.211

[32] Greenberg MS. Interpretation of transcranial dopplerography in vascular spasm. In: Handbook of Neurosurgery. New York: THIEME VERLAGSGRUPPE; 2006. p. 793

[33] Polushin AY, Odinak MM, Voznyuk IA, Yanishevsky SN. Extended Doppler monitoring of cerebral blood flow in different subtypes of ischemic stroke. Annals of Clinical and Experimental Neurology. 2015;**9**(3): 26-33

[34] Polushin AY, Voznyuk A. The rate of cerebral blood flow – a prognostic marker and the purpose of monitoring in acute cerebral ischemia. Medline. 2014;**15**(1):175-184

[35] Voznyuk A, Yu PA, Stepanov E. Is. Quantitative assessment of ultrasound parameters of cerebral blood flow (norm and value). Regional Blood Circulation and Microcirculation. 2013;**12**(4):30-40

[36] Macdonald RL. Management of cerebral vasospasm. Neurosurgical Review. 2006;**29**:179-193

[37] Gonzalez NR, Boscardin WJ, Glenn T, Vinuela F, Martin NA. Vasospasm probability index: A combination of transcranial Doppler velocities, cerebral blood flow, and clinical risk factors to predict cerebral vasospasm after aneurismal subarachnoid hemorrhage. Journal of Neurosurgery. 2007;**107**:1101-1112

[38] Harrod CG, Bendok BR, Batjer HH. Prediction of cerebral vasospasm in patients presenting with aneurismal subarachnoid hemorrhage: A review. Neurosurgery. 2005;**56**:633-654

[39] Macdonald RL, Rosengart A, Huo D, Karrison T. Factors associated with the development of vasospasm after planned surgical treatment of aneurismal subarachnoid hemorrhage. Journal of Neurosurgery. 2003;**99**: 644-652

[40] Gurusinghe NT, Richardson AE. The value of computerized tomography in aneurismal subarachnoid hemorrhage. Journal of Neurosurgery. 1984;**60**:763-770

[41] Nestor RG, Boscardin WJ, Glenn T, Vinuela F, Martin NA. Vasospasm probability index: A combination of transcranial Doppler velocities, cerebral blood flow, and clinical risk factors to predict cerebral vasospasm after aneurysmal subarachnoid hemorrhage. Journal of Neurosurgery. 2007;**107**(6): 1101-1112

[42] Konovalov AN, Krylov VV, Filatov YM, et al. Recommendation protocol for the management of patients with subarachnoid hemorrhage due to rupture of cerebral aneurysms. Questions of Neurosurgery. 2006;**3**:3-10

[43] Reimers V, Cernetti S, Sacca S, et al. Stenting of the carotid artery with the protection of the cerebral filter. Journal of Angiology Vascular Surgery. 2002;**8**(3):57-62

[44] Song JK, Kakayorin ED, Campbell MS, et al. Intracranial balloon angioplasty in acute terminal occlusions of the internal carotid artery. American Journal of Neuroradiology. 2002;**23**(8): 1308-1312

[45] Fisher CM, Kistler JP, Davis JM. Relation of cerebral vasospasm to subarachnoid hemorrhage visualized by computerized tomographic scanning. Neurosurgery. 1980;**6**:1-9

[46] Kistler JP, Crowell RM, Davis KR, Heros R, Ojemann RG, Zervas T, et al. The relation of cerebral vasospasm to the extent and location of subarachnoid blood visualized by CT scan: A prospective study. Neurology. 1983;**33**(4):424-436

[47] Rosen DS, McDonald RL, Huo D, et al. Intraventricular hemorrhage from a ruptured aneurysm: Clinical characteristics, complications and outcomes in a large, prospective multicenter study. Journal of Neurosurgery. 2007;**107**(2):261-265

[48] Nomura Y, Kawaguchi M, Yoshitani K, et al. Retrospective analysis of predictors of cerebral vasospasm after ruptured cerebral aneurysm surgery: Influence of the location of subarachnoid blood. Journal of Anesthesia. 2010;**24**:1-6. DOI: 10.1007/s00540-009-0836-2

[49] Mohsen F, Pomonis S, Illingworth R. Prediction of delayed cerebral ischaemia after subarachnoid haemorrhage by computed tomography. Journal of Neurology, Neurosurgery, and Psychiatry. 1984;**47**:1197-1202

[50] Brouwers PJ, Dippel DW, Vermeulen M, Lindsay KW, Hasan D, van Gijn J. Amount of blood on computed tomography as an independent predictor after aneurysm rupture. Stroke. 1993;**24**:809-814

[51] Reilly C, Amidei C, Tolentino J, Jahromi BS, Macdonald RL. Clot volume and clearance rate as independent predictors of vasospasm after aneurismal subarachnoid hemorrhage. Journal of Neurosurgery. 2004;**101**:255-261

[52] Hijdra A, van Gijn J, Nagelkerke NJ, Vermelen M, van Crevel H. Prediction of delayed cerebral ischemia, rebleeding, and outcome after aneurismal subarachnoid hemorrhage. Stroke. 1988;**19**:1250-1256

[53] Claassen J, Bernardini GL, Kreiter K, Bates J, Du YE, Copeland D, et al. Effect of cisternal and ventricular blood on risk of delayed cerebral ischemia after subarachnoid hemorrhage: The Fisher scale revisited. Stroke. 2001;**32**:2012-2020

[54] Peerless SJ, Fox AJ, Komatsu K, Hunter IG. Angiographic study of vasospasm following subarachnoid hemorrhage in monkeys. Stroke. 1982;**13**:473-479

[55] Bunc G, Kovacic S, Strnad S. The influence of noradrenergic blockade on vasospasm and the quality of cerebral dopamine beta-hydroxylase following subarachnoid haemorrhage in rabbits. Wiener Klinische Wochenschrift. 2003;**115**:652-659

[56] Morooka H. Cerebral arterial spasm. I. Adrenergic mechanism in experimental cerebral vasospasm. Acta Medica Okayama. 1978;**32**:23-37

[57] Lobato R, Marin J, Salaices M, Burgos J, Rivilla F, Garcia AG. Effect of experimental subarachnoid hemorrhage on the adrenergic innervation of cerebral arteries. Journal of Neurosurgery. 1980;**53**:477-479

[58] Kovacic S, Bunc G, Ravnik J. Correspondence between the time course of cerebral vasospasm and the level of cerebral dopamine-beta-hydroxylase in rabbits. Autonomic Neuroscience. 2006;**130**:28-31

[59] Hirashima Y, Takashima S, Matsumura N, Kurimoto M, Origasa H, Endo S. Right sylvian fissure subarachnoid hemorrhage has electrocardiographic consequences. Stroke. 2001;**32**:2278-2281

[60] Kato H, Kawaguchi M, Inoue S, Hirai K, Furuya H. The effects of beta-adrenoceptor antagonists on proinflammatory cytokine concentrations after subarachnoid hemorrhage in rats. Anesthesia and Analgesia. 2009;**108**(1):288-295

[61] Savvina IA, Cherebillo VY, Zabrodskaya YM, Petrova AO, Sergeev AV, Paltsev AA, et al. The intraoperative prophylaxis of local ischemical brain damage in neurosurgical patients with cerebral

aneurysm. Pirogov Journal of Surgery. 2019;**5**:65-71

[62] Kondratyev AN, Tsentsiper LM, Kondratyeva EA, Nazarov RV. Neurovegetative stabilization as a pathogenetic therapy of brain injury. Anesthesiology and Reanimatology. 2014;**1**:82-84

[63] Shevelev OA, Grechko AV, Petrova MV, et al. Theraputic Hypothermia. Moscow: Publishing House of Russian University of Friendship of Peoples; 2019. p. 256

Section 3

Intervention and Rehabilitation

Chapter 7

Thrombolysis in Acute Stroke

Mustafa Çetiner

Abstract

The first step in stroke care is early detection of stroke patients and recanalization of the occluded vessel. Rapid and effective revascularization is the cornerstone of acute ischemic stroke management. Intravenous thrombolysis is the only approved pharmacological reperfusion therapy for patients with acute ischemic stroke. Patient selection criteria based on patient characteristics, time, clinical findings and advanced neuroimaging techniques have positively affected treatment outcomes. Recent studies show that the presence of salvageable brain tissue can extend the treatment window for intravenous thrombolysis and that these patients can be treated safely. Recent evidence provides stronger support for another thrombolytic agent, tenecteplase, as an alternative to alteplase. Endovascular thrombectomy is not a contraindication for intravenous thrombolysis. Evidence shows that the bridging approach provides better clinical outcomes. It is seen that intravenous thrombolysis is beneficial in stroke patients, whose symptom onset is not known, after the presence of penumbra tissue is revealed by advanced neuroimaging techniques. Reperfusion therapy with intravenous thrombolysis is beneficial in selected pregnant stroke patients. Pregnancy should not be an absolute contraindication for thrombolysis therapy. This chapter aims to review only the current evaluation of intravenous thrombolytic therapy, one of the reperfusion therapies applied in the acute phase of stroke.

Keywords: acute strokes, collateral flow, ischemic penumbra, thrombolysis, reperfusion

1. Introduction

Stroke is a very common global health problem causing mortality and long-term disability [1]. It is a devastating disease and a significant economic burden on society [1–4]. It is an infarction of the central nervous system and approximately 85% of all strokes are ischemic in nature [4, 5].

For this reason, stroke treatment has a narrow time frame in the acute process, and therefore is very important. Acute ischemic stroke (AIS) is defined by loss of neurological function as a result of arterial occlusion and sudden loss of blood flow in an area of the brain. It occurs as a result of thrombosis or embolism [6–8]. After the occlusion, infarct tissue forms in the center of the irrigation area of the vessel within minutes. In its periphery, there is a reversible ischemic area that can be saved by recanalization of the vessel called the penumbra, where cell death has not yet occurred thanks to the collateral flow. This blood flow is usually weak and can sustain the penumbral region only for a limited time. Unless recanalization is provided, the region is doomed to progress to infarction [9].

Purpose in the treatment of acute ischemic stroke is to recanalize the occluded vessel as soon as possible and to ensure reperfusion in this region without cell death, because more irreversible cell damage occurs with each passing minute [10]. Collateral flow and reperfusion time are the most important factors affecting the outcome [9]. The emergence of effective pharmacological and endovascular reperfusion treatment strategies has revolutionized the treatment of stroke over the past two decades. Today, death and disability in stroke can be significantly reduced with intravenous thrombo-lytic therapy (IVT) followed by endovascular recanalization treatments [11, 12].

2. Neuroimaging in acute stroke

Neuroimaging is essential for the diagnosis and treatment of stroke. Since whether the etiology of the patient presenting with the stroke clinic is ischemic or hemorrhagic origin cannot be distinguished, urgent brain imaging is needed. Non-contrast brain computed tomography (NCCT) is recommended as soon as possible (ideally within 20 min) [8, 12].

CT is sufficient to decide on thrombolysis in acute strokes within 4.5 h after the onset of the symptom. It remains the only mandatory radiological examina-tion before IVT [12, 13]. Noninvasive intracranial vascular imaging should also be performed in patients with suspected large vessel occlusion and who may require endovascular recanalization therapy, without delaying IV thrombolytic therapy [8, 13]. Diffusion-weighted imaging (DWI) can be used because it shows the infarct tissue most accurately. Stroke patients with large infarct volumes (>100 ml) at baseline are at increased risk of bleeding after reperfusion [7]. A study with uncer-tain onset time reported a better functional improvement with IV thrombolytic therapy based on the discordance between diffusion and FLAIR-weighted magnetic resonance imaging (MRI) [14].

CT and MR perfusion have been used in recent studies to select patients who may benefit from treatments in stroke patients outside the typical time windows for reperfusion therapy (4.5 h for intravenous alteplase versus 6 h for endovascu-lar therapy) [15–17]. Perfusion imaging is used to evaluate the amount and timing of blood flow to specific areas of the brain. It gives us information about the infarct area and penumbra. Thus, it contributes to better patient selection, higher rates of reperfusion therapy, and better functional results in more stroke patients [15, 16, 18]. Perfusion studies present various parameters such as cerebral blood volume and flow (CBV and CBF), mean transit time (MTT), and time to peak (Tmax). CBV indicates irreversibly damaged brain tissue while Tmax and MTT indicate hypoperfused tissue at risk of infarction [19–21]. These studies may also be helpful in distinguishing acute cerebrovascular events from common stroke mimics [22]. Therefore, further imaging is critical in identifying the patient profile that will benefit most from endovascular thrombectomy (EVT) and IVT. Today, CT and MR-based advanced imaging have become ideal acute stroke imag-ing tools and have been considered the standard in many stroke centers around the world [13, 20, 23].

3. Acute reperfusion strategies

The main purpose of AIS treatment is to save brain tissue at risk for ischemia by recanalizing occluded cerebral arteries and providing reperfusion. IV throm-bolysis and EVT have been proven to improve neurological outcomes. Now, the use of multimodal CT and MRI is going beyond the known therapeutic time window by applying individualized treatment to appropriate stroke patients [17, 18, 21, 22, 24].

3.1 Alteplase

Recombinant human tissue plasminogen activator (r-tPA) converts plasmino-gen to plasmin and cleaves the formed thrombus. IV alteplase has a half-life of less than 5 min and is cleared primarily by the liver [25]. In 1995, a study of The National Institute of Neurological Disorders and Stroke (NINDS) demonstrated the effectiveness of IV thrombolytic therapy in patients with acute ischemic stroke within 3 h after the symptom onset [26]. IV thrombolytic therapy has been shown to be beneficial among patients of different age groups, different types of ischemic stroke, and stroke severity [27]. Later studies extended the treatment window to 4.5 h [28].

3.1.1 Efficiency

Results from major randomized trials of IV r-tPA (alteplase) for AIS showed a significant reduction in disability. The benefit from IV thrombolysis is much greater in the first 90 min from the onset of symptoms [9]. To achieve excellent functional outcome [modified Ranking Scale (mRS $\leq$ 1)], the number of patients required to be treated increases from 4.5 within the first 90 min to 15 between 3 and 4.5 h [29]. The diminished effect is related to the loss of salvaged penumbral tissue over time [10]. The susceptibility of thrombus to lysis may also decrease over time, which may reduce the effectiveness of treatment in late administration [30]. Recent evidence suggests that there may be patients with ongoing ischemic penumbra on perfusion imaging and that IV r-tPA may still be beneficial up to 9 h from the symptom onset [31].

3.1.2 Risks

The most feared complication of IV thrombolysis is symptomatic intracerebral hemorrhage (sICH). The current definition of sICH requires that the hemorrhage reach at least 30% of the infarct volume and cause a mass effect. Accordingly, data suggest that the risk of sICH is 1.7% [11, 32]. Intracerebral hemorrhage occurs mostly in the first 12 h. It is associated with age, diabetes, severe hyperglycemia, uncontrolled hypertension, and greater hypodensity at baseline CT scan, stroke severity, and concomitant antiplatelet therapy. Patients with cerebral microhemor-rhage may also be at increased risk of sICH. When the patient is diagnosed with sICH after thrombolysis is made, blood pressure regulation should be established immedi-ately. Cryoprecipitate should then be given until fibrinogen levels return to normal. Tranexamic acid or aminocaproic acid can also be used in therapy [9, 13, 33].

Orolingual angioedema occurs in approximately 1% of patients (5% if taking angiotensin converting enzyme inhibitors). Treatment includes diphenhydramine (50 mg IV), ranitidine (50 mg IV), and dexamethasone (10 mg IV) [9]. Icatibant (a bradykinin receptor antagonist) can be used in severe cases to avoid the need for intubation [34, 35].

Evidence-based current indications and contraindications of IV r-tPA in acute stroke are presented in **Table 1** [9, 12].

3.2 Tenecteplase

Tenecteplase (TNK) is a newer thrombolytic agent with some pharmacological advantages over alteplase. It is infused faster and is cheaper. It is a variant of r-tPA with a longer half-life, higher affinity for fibrin, and administered as an IV bolus (0.4 mg/kg, maximum 40 mg dose) only once [36]. Randomized clinical trial results demonstrated that tenecteplase is safe and effective in stroke patients. It was

Indications	Contraindications
• Clinical diagnosis of ischemic stroke	• Acute intracerebral, subarachnoid, subdural hemorrhage
• Age: 18	• Presence of extensive hypodensity in CT
• Time from the stroke onset? 4.5 h	• Systolic blood pressure > 185 mm/Hg or diastolic blood pressure > 110 mm/Hg and uncontrolled hypertension
• Absence of bleeding on entry CT scan	• Thrombocytopenia (<100.000/mm^3)
• Wake-up stroke with diffusion-weighted imaging-FLAIR mismatch on MRI	• INR > 1.7, aPTT >40 s
	• Gastrointestinal bleeding in the last 3 weeks
	• Cranial/spinal surgery in the last 3 months
	• Cranial/spinal trauma in the past 3 months
	• Ischemic stroke in the last 3 months
	• History of intracranial bleeding
	• Active internal bleeding
	• Bleeding diathesis
	• Aortic dissection
	• Infective endocarditis
	• Intracranial intraaxial tumor
	• Use of NOAC (non-vitamin K antagonist oral anti-coagulant) in the last 48 h
	• Low-molecular-weight heparin full treatment dose within previous 24 h

CT: computed brain tomography.

Table 1.
Indications and contraindications for the use of alteplase in acute ischemic stroke.

observed that it had higher reperfusion rates compared to alteplase in patients with large vessel occlusion [36, 37].

The NOR-TEST randomized trial evaluated the safety and efficacy of 0.4 mg/kg tenecteplase (max. 40 mg) versus standard dose alteplase over a 4.5 h time frame. The rates of sICH and functional recovery in 3 months were similar in both groups [38].

In the EXTEND-IA TNK Part 2 study, it was reported that increasing the dose from 0.25 mg/kg to 0.40 mg in patients with large vessel occlusion before endovascular treatment was not an advantage [39]. In case of implementation of tenecteplase, since many patients are transferred between hospitals for treatment, a single bolus administration will facilitate the transport process and ensure that the full dose of the thrombolytic agent can be administered [37, 40].

Current guidelines indicate tenecteplase as an alternative to r-tPA only in patients with mild stroke [41]. A meta-analysis of five randomized studies (1585 patients (828 TNK, 757 alteplase) provided strong evidence that TNK is noninferior to alteplase in functional improvement in the treatment of acute ischemic stroke. These findings provide stronger support for considering TNK as an alternative to alteplase [42].

3.3 Low-dose IV thrombolytic therapy

IV rtPA at standard dose (0.9 mg/kg–90 mg maximum dose) is effective in all stroke types [26, 43–45]. The most feared complication among clinicians is sICH [28].

Therefore, low-dose thrombolysis applications have come to the fore. In the non-randomized Japanese Alteplase Clinical Trial (J-ACT) [46], in which 0.6 mg/kg (maximum 60 mg) r-tPA therapy was administered to patients in the first 3 h of acute ischemic stroke, compared to the standard dose, equivalent clinical results and a reduced risk of sICH were found. After J-ACT and other reports in Japan [47, 48], the use of 0.6 mg/kg alteplase as a treatment regimen in acute ischemic stroke was approved by the Japanese Pharmaceuticals Safety Authority [49].

Also, in a comprehensive meta-analysis study, it was reported that low-dose rtPA is effective and more reliable, and low-dose tPA is recommended in patients with acute ischemic stroke [50]. However, in another randomized study (3310 patients), comparing these two doses on mostly Asian patients, although the risk of symptomatic intracerebral hemorrhage in the low dose group decreased from 2–1%, low-dose thrombolytic therapy could not be shown to be effective [51].

In a retrospective study of 1486 patients by Zhao et al., there was no significant difference in rates of good clinical outcome between the low-dose and standard-dose groups (36.1% vs. 37.6%; p = 0.89). However, the incidence of sICH in the low-dose group was significantly lower than in the standard-dose group (2.2% vs. 5.9%. p = 0.001). The results showed that low-dose thrombolysis was safer in acute stroke [52].

In a meta-analysis that included retrospective, prospective, observational, and randomized controlled trials, the low-dose strategy was also found to be as effective as standard-dose tPA (good functional outcome: 43.4% vs. 45.4%; p = 0.38). There was also no significant difference between the rates of sICH (4.2% vs. 4.9%; p = 0.94). This meta-analysis study also showed that AIS patients receiving low-dose IV-rtPA had similar efficacy and safety compared to those receiving standard-dose IV-rtPA [53].

In the treatment of acute ischemic stroke, the licensed dose for alteplase in Japan is 0.6 mg/kg, and in all treatment guidelines except Japan, it is recommended that 10% is bolused, followed by the remaining 90%, with a total dose of 0.9 mg/kg (maximum 90 mg), to be administered as an infusion in 1 h [40].

3.4 Combination of intravenous thrombolytic therapy and endovascular treatment

EVT has become the standard treatment for patients with acute ischemic stroke caused by major vessel occlusions. EVT therapy is not a contraindication for IV thrombolysis. IVT prior to endovascular therapy can rapidly recanalize the occluded vessel, thus eliminating the need for EVT and shortening the ischemia time. Moreover, even if it does not dissolve the thrombus, it alters the clot structure, making it more susceptible to endovascular removal of the thrombus. The newly embolized thrombi in the distal vessels that may occur at the end of the EVT procedure generally cannot be accessed by mechanical thrombectomy. IVT can also successfully resolve these thrombi. However, IVT application before EVT may cause adverse effects. Initiation of endovascular therapy may be delayed if the time taken to initiate IVT is not done in parallel with the steps required to initiate EVT. IVT causes partial disintegration of the thrombus, resulting in distal emboli. Access to these areas may not be possible with endovascular intervention. Thus, it can turn a treatable thrombus into an incurable condition. In addition, the combined use of EVT and IVT causes increased treatment costs [54].

In observational and meta-analysis studies, it has been reported that the bridging treatment approach provides better clinical results [55–57].

Recent evidence contributes to the fact that EVT alone is non-inferior to the functional outcomes achieved with combined IVT + EVT for patients with large vessel occlusion with acute stroke [58, 59].

Currently, bridging therapy is recommended in large vessel occlusions with anterior circulation in current guidelines. However, this should not delay the initiation of endovascular treatment [41, 60].

4. Special situations

Evidence is insufficient to determine the treatment approach in some specific clinical situations. Until definitive data are available, individual factors should be considered in the approach to these patients and clinical experience should be taken into account.

4.1 Intravenous thrombolysis in patients with acute ischemic stroke with unknown onset time

Wake-up stroke (WUS) is a stroke whose exact onset time is unknown. They constitute 20% of all ischemic strokes. Patients with acute ischemic stroke whose neurological deficit is recognized upon awakening and whose onset is unknown pose a particular challenge for the clinician. Until recently, WUS was considered a contraindication to reperfusion therapy due to its unknown onset time and intracerebral hemorrhage that may be associated with thrombolytic therapy. The clinical efficacy of reperfusion therapy in selected patients with WUS was displayed by demonstrating the presence of salvageable brain tissue in advanced brain imaging [61]. Also, in a recent meta-analysis study (77,398 patients), stroke patients with unknown symptom onset were proven to be safely and effectively treated with IV-tPA guided by imaging evaluation [62]. In the WAKE-UP randomized study, IV thrombolytic therapy was administered to acute stroke patients. In these patients, onset time was unknown, and it was based on the discrepancy between diffusion and FLAIR-weighted MRI in the ischemia region. The treatment group showed a better functional recovery at 90 days compared to the placebo [14]. The use of WAKE-UP study criteria (DWI—FLAIR mismatch) to select patients in symptomatic strokes for intravenous alteplase treatment was recommended as class IIa in the 2019 AHA/ASA guidelines [12]. ESO IVT guidelines also advocate thrombolytic therapy in patients with DWI/FLAIR mismatch in recovery strokes [63].

In the EXTEND randomized trial, it was shown that if there is evidence of salvageable brain tissue that has not yet been transformed into infarct, with perfusion imaging between 4.5 h and 9.0 h (within 9 h from the midpoint of sleep on wake-up stroke) from the last time the patients were seen well, the treatment window could be expanded andbetter functional results were obtained than the standard treatment. Symptomatic intracerebral hemorrhage rates were similar to patients who received IV thrombolytic therapy in the classical time window [17].

The THAWS study evaluated whether low-dose alteplase 0.6 mg/kg was effective and safe for stroke of unknown onset. There was no difference in functional outcomes when compared with the placebo group [64].

In another randomized trial (ECASS-4), administering intravenous alteplase to patients selected with advanced brain imaging following 4.5–9 h after the onset of symptoms did not provide a significant benefit over the placebo [65].

For WUS patients and the ones with unknown symptom onset, IV thrombolysis is beneficial only after the presence of penumbra tissue is revealed by advanced neuroimaging techniques. Patients with small infarct core and large penumbra tissue are selected prior to IV thrombolysis application. It has been reported that IV thrombolytic therapy in these patients provides a decrease in infarct volume and better functional results without an increase in bleeding risk in recovery strokes [66].

Clinical trial	Patients, (n)	Imaging modality	Time window (h)	sICH	Outcome
ECASS-4	119	MRI/MRP ischemic core <70 ml, PWI lesion minimum volume of 20 ml	4.5–9	1.6%	No significant difference between functional outcomes
WAKE-UP	503	DWI-positive FLAIR negative	Unknown time of symptom onset	2%	90 day mRS < 2 alteplase 53.3%; placebo 41.8%; p = 0.02
EXTEND	225	MRI/MRP CT/CTP ischemic core <70 ml and mismatch volume > 10 ml	4.5–9	6.2%	90 day mRS < 2; alteplase 35.4%; placebo 29.5%; p = 0.04
THAWS	131	DWI-positive FLAIR negative	4.5–12	1.4%	90 day mRS < 2; alteplase 47%; placebo 48%; p = 0.89

CT: computed brain tomography, CTP: CT perfusion, DWI: diffusion-weighted imaging, MRI: magnetic resonance imaging, MRP: MR perfusion, sICH: symptomatic intracerebral hemorrhage.

Table 2.
Summary of randomized controlled trials of late (beyond 4.5 h) IV thrombolysis.

However, imaging-based late thrombolytic treatment recommendations are not commonly at the level of guideline [60].

A summary of imaging-based IV thrombolysis studies in wake-up strokes beyond the therapeutic window and strokes of unknown symptom onset is presented in **Table 2**.

An 84-year-old male patient with a wake-up stroke, whose symptoms were noticed 5 h after his last known well-being, had NIHSS:20. Significant penumbra was detected as a result of MRI-based multimodal imaging. Clinical and advanced imaging findings for IV thrombolysis therapy meet the patient selection criteria in the WAKE-UP and EXTEND studies. In the 6th hour of the clinic IV, thrombolysis was started and successful recanalization was achieved (**Figure 1**).

4.2 Stroke in pregnancy

The incidence of stroke in pregnancy is about 9–34 per 100,000 deliveries. Strokes are three times more common in pregnant women than in non-pregnant individuals aged 15–44 [67, 68]. Causes of pregnancy-related stroke include pregnancy-specific causes such as preeclampsia/eclampsia, postpartum angiopathy, amniotic fluid embolism and postpartum cardiomyopathy, and other causes like hypertension, diabetes, vasculitis, arteriovenous malformations or aneurysms [69].

4.2.1 Brain imaging in pregnancy stroke

MRI should be the first-line imaging modality of choice in pregnancy as it does not expose the pregnant woman to radiation. Up to 3 tesla MRI has no harmful effects on the fetus [70].

Access to CT is easier. Therefore, it is also preferred during pregnancy in acute neurological conditions. The fetal radiation dose on non-contrast CT is approximately 5% of the naturally occurring radiation dose during a pregnancy (on average, this is 0.5–1.0 mGy) [68]. Studies report that a dose of fetal radiation less than 0.1 Gy (100 mGy) has no risk of adverse effect in humans [68, 71]. The radiation effect on the fetus will be minimized by using a 0.5 mm thick lead apron during the shooting [68].

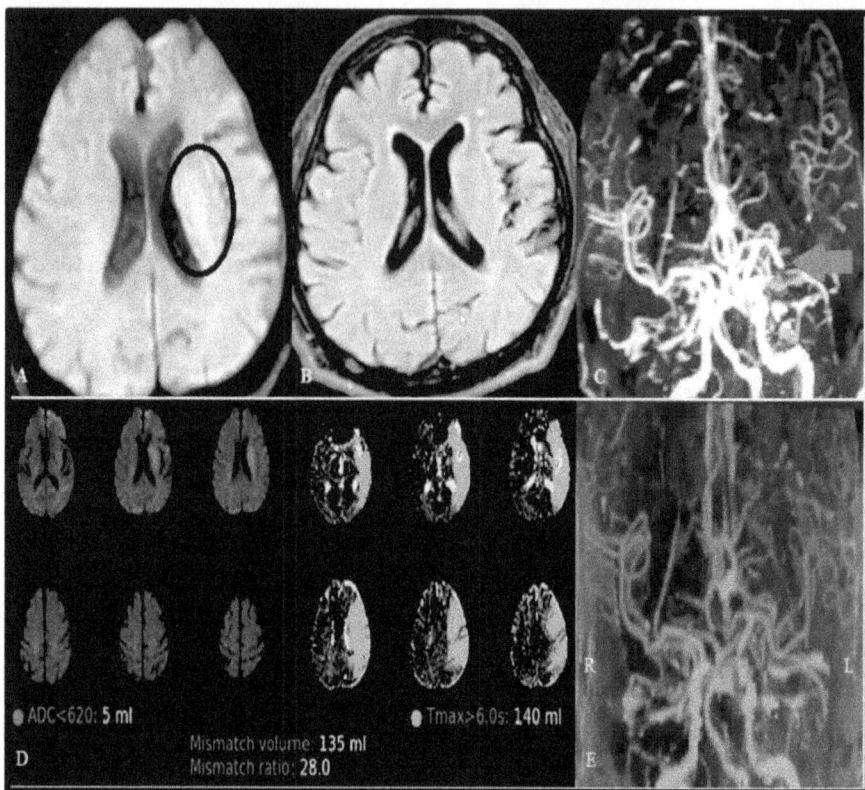

Figure 1.
(A) Hyperintensity in the right lentiform nucleus on diffusion MRI (black circle). (B) The infarct does not appear to be reflected in Flair MRI. (C) Left MCA M1 segment is occluded in CTA (red arrow). (D) In MR perfusion imaging calculated with RAPID automatic software program, infarct volume: 5 ml, Tmax > 6 s, volume (critical hypoperfused area): 140 ml, mismatch volume: 135 ml. Mismatch ratio: 28. (E) Left MCA was recanalized after IV thrombolysis (Istinye University Liv Hospital Neurology Clinic Archive-Istanbul/Turkey).

4.2.2 Thrombolysis in pregnancy

Alteplase and tenecteplase, in animal studies, are large molecules that do not cross the placenta and are not teratogenic at stroke treatment doses [72]. There are no randomized controlled trials of the treatment of acute stroke with thrombolysis or mechanical thrombectomy to guide decision-making in the pregnant population [72–74]. Successful reperfusion with IV thrombolysis and good clinical results were reported in pregnant acute stroke patients in case series. With the help of advanced neuroimaging techniques, Erin et al. also reported good clinical outcome with successful reperfusion with IV rt-PA in a pregnant patient with acute ischemic stroke outside the therapeutic window (>4.5/<9 h) [75].

According to the (AHA/ASA) guidelines, treatment of acute ischemic stroke with intravenous alteplase during pregnancy is recommended when the expected benefit of treatment for moderate to severe stroke outweighs (class IIb) [41].

The dose of IV thrombolysis for a pregnant patient with acute stroke should be calculated considering the pre-pregnancy or early pregnancy weight. Close monitoring of the pregnant patient during IV thrombolysis is important because of the risk of placental abruption. Blood pressure should be closely monitored during IV thrombolysis. During pregnancy, it is recommended to maintain it between 140 and

160/90–110 mmHg during tPA therapy. Intravenous nicardipine and labetalol are recommended agents for BP control [76].

Reperfusion therapy with IV thrombolysis in acute stroke in pregnant women remains controversial, but pregnancy should not be a contraindication for mechanical thrombectomy and tPA therapy in selected patients.

4.3 Thrombolysis In posterior circulation stroke

IVT is the standard treatment for both anterior circulation ischemic strokes (ACIS) and posterior circulation ischemic strokes (PCIS) [77, 78]. In PCIS, the rate of intravenous thrombolysis administered is between 5% and 19% [77]. Basilar artery occlusion (BAO) is a devastating disease causing high mortality and serious disability. Even among patients treated with reperfusion strategies, mortality is high [79, 80]. Therefore, clinicians consider that these patients should be treated with aggressive treatment approaches and go beyond the reperfusion treatment window [79, 81].

The rate of sICH in PCIs after IVT is between 0 and 6.9%. Good functional outcome is reported in 38–49% (mRS 0–1) of the patients with PCIS. Better clinical outcomes are seen more often in patients with PCIS than the ones with ACIS. There is no significant difference between mortality rates. Results from retrospective clinical studies and case series report that IVT is safer for use in PCIS than ACIS [81].

5. Conclusion

AIS is a medical emergency where every minute counts. Rapid recanalization of the clogged vessel is the most effective treatment. IV thrombolysis is effective and safe in suitable candidates. IV thrombolysis is one of the two reperfusion strategies in acute stroke. Unless there is an absolute contraindication, eligible patients with acute stroke should be treated with IV r-tPA. Even in severe strokes, reperfusion can improve neurological dysfunction and enable patients to live independently. In studies, the time from stroke onset to treatment time is critical, although advanced neuroimaging techniques identify patients who will benefit most from intravenous thrombolysis and enable stroke patients whose onset time cannot be determined to be treated with intravenous thrombolysis. From this perspective, more efforts should be made to ensure that more patients reach treatment faster. Much better clinical results can be achieved with the continuous education of the society and stroke personnel, the rapid assessment of patients with a multidisciplinary approach in the emergency department, early recognition of stroke patients, and the best management of in-hospital and out-of-hospital stroke algorithms. The expansion of mobile stroke units, experienced clinicians and stroke centers will contribute to this issue.

Conflict of interest

The author declare no conflict of interest.

Author details

Mustafa Çetiner
Department of Neurology, Faculty of Medicine, Kütahya Health Sciences
University, Kütahya, Turkey

*Address all correspondence to: drcetiner76@gmail.com

IntechOpen

References

[1] Saver JL, Hankey GJ. Stroke Prevention and Treatment. 2nd ed. United Kingdom: Cambridge University; 2021. 570 p. DOI: 10.1017/9781316286234

[2] Lopez AD, Mathers CD, Ezzati M, et al. Global and regional burden of disease and risk factors, 2001: Systematic analysis of population health data. Lancet. 2006;**367**:1747-1757. DOI: 10.1016/S0140-6736(06)68770-9

[3] Feigin VL, Forouzanfar MH, Krishnamurthi R, et al. Global and regional burden of stroke during 1990-2010: Findings from the Global Burden of Disease Study 2010. Lancet. 2014;**383**:245-254. DOI: 10.1016/s0140-6736(13)61953-4

[4] Mikulik R, Wahlgren N. Treatment of acute stroke: An update. Journal of Internal Medicine. 2015;**278**:145-165. DOI: 10.1111/joim.12387

[5] Benjamin EJ, Muntner P, Alonso A. Heart disease and stroke statistics-2019 update: A report from the American Heart Association. Circulation. 2019;**139**(10):e56-e528. DOI: 10.1161/CIR.0000000000000659

[6] Saver JL. Time is brain—Quantified. Stroke. 2006;**37**(1):263-266. DOI: 10.1161/01.STR.0000196957.55928.ab

[7] Kamalian S, Lev MH. Stroke imaging. Radiologic Clinics of North America. 2019;**57**:717-732. DOI: 10.1016/j.rcl.2019.02.001

[8] Phipps MS, Cronin CA. Management of acute ischemic stroke. BMJ. 2020;**368**:l6983. DOI: 10.1136/bmj.l6983

[9] Rabinstein AA. Update on treatment of acute ischemic stroke. Continuum (Minneap Minn). 2020;**26**(2):268-286. DOI: 10.1212/CON.0000000000000840

[10] Campbell BCV, De Silva DA, Macleod MR, et al. Ischaemic stroke. Nature Reviews Disease Primers. 2019;**5**:70. DOI: 10.1038/s41572-019-0118-8

[11] Campbell BC. Advances in stroke medicine. Medical Journal of Australia. 2019;**210**:367-374. DOI: 10.5694/mja2.50137

[12] Powers WJ, Rabinstein AA, Ackerson T, et al. Guidelines for the early management of patients with acute ischemic stroke: 2019 update to the 2018 guidelines for the early management of acute ischemic stroke: A guideline for healthcare professionals from the American Heart Association/American Stroke Association. Stroke. 2019;**50**(12):e344-e418. DOI: 10.1161/STR.0000000000000211

[13] Morotti A, Poli L, Costa P. Acute stroke. Seminars in Neurology. 2019;**39**:61-72. DOI: 10.1055/s-0038-1676992

[14] Thomalla G, Simonsen CZ, Boutitie F, et al. MRI-guided thrombolysis for stroke with unknown time of onset. The New England Journal of Medicine. 2018;**379**:611-622. DOI: 10.1056/NEJMoa1804355

[15] Albers GW, Marks MP, Kemp S, et al. Thrombectomy for stroke at 6 to 16 hours with selection by perfusion imaging. The New England Journal of Medicine. 2018;**378**:708-718. DOI: 10.1056/NEJMoa1713973

[16] Nogueira RG, Jadhav AP, Haussen DC, et al. Thrombectomy 6 to 24 hours after stroke with a mismatch between deficit and infarct. The New England Journal of Medicine. 2018;**378**:11-21. DOI: 10.1056/NEJMoa1706442

[17] Ma H, Campbell BCV, Parsons MW, et al. Thrombolysis guided by perfusion imaging up to 9 hours after onset of stroke. The New England Journal of

Medicine. 2019;**380**:1795-1803. DOI: 10.1056/NEJMoa1813046

[18] Ryu WHA, Avery MB, Dharampal N, et al. Utility of perfusion imaging in acute stroke treatment: A systematic review and meta-analysis. Journal of NeuroInterventional Surgery. 2017;**9**:1012-1016. DOI: 10.1136/neurintsurg-2016-012751

[19] Vilela P, Rowley HA. Brain ischemia: CT and MRI techniques in acute ischemic stroke. European Journal of Radiology. 2017;**96**:162-172. DOI: 10.1016/j.ejrad.2017.08.014

[20] Rudkin S, Cerejo R, Tayal A, et al. Imaging of acute ischemic stroke. Emergency Radiology. 2018;**25**(06):659-672. DOI: 10.1007/s10140-018-1623-x

[21] Campbell BCV, Parsons MW. Imaging selection for acute strokes intervention. International Journal of Stroke. 2018;**13**(06):554-567. DOI: 10.1177/1747493018765235

[22] Campbell BCV, Weir L, Desmond PM, et al. CT perfusion improves diagnostic accuracy and confidence in acute ischaemic stroke. Journal of Neurology, Neurosurgery, and Psychiatry. 2013;**84**(06):613-618. DOI: 10.1136/jnnp-2012-303752

[23] Hollist M, Morgan L, Cabatbat R, et al. Acute stroke management: Overview and recent updates. Aging and Disease. 2021;**12**(4):1000-1009. DOI: 10.14336/AD.2021.0311

[24] Etherton MR, Gadhia RR, Schwamm LH. Thrombolysis beyond 4.5 h in acute ischemic stroke. Current Neurology and Neuroscience Reports. 2020;**20**(8):35. DOI: 10.1007/s11910-020-01055-1

[25] StatPearls [Internet]. Treasure Island (FL): StatPearls Publishing; 2021. Editorial Board. Available from: https://www.ncbi.nlm.nih.gov/books/NBK431128/

[26] National Institute of Neurological Disorders and Stroke rt-PA Stroke Study Group. Tissue plasminogen activator for acute ischemic stroke. The New England Journal of Medicine. 1995;**333**:1581-1587. DOI: 10.1056/NEJM199512143332401

[27] Liaw N, Liebeskind D. Emerging therapies in acute ischemic stroke. F1000Research. 2020;**9**:546. DOI: 10.12688/f1000research.21100.1

[28] Emberson J, Lees KR, Lyden P, et al. Effect of treatment delay, age, and stroke severity on the effects of intravenous thrombolysis with alteplase for acute ischaemic stroke: A meta-analysis of individual patient data from randomised trials. Lancet. 2014;**384**: 1929-1935. DOI: 10.1016/S0140-6736(14)60584-5

[29] Lees KR, Bluhmki E, von Kummer R, et al. Time to treatment with intravenous alteplase and outcome in stroke: An updated pooled analysis of ECASS, ATLANTIS, NINDS, and EPITHET trials. Lancet. 2010;**375**:1695-1703. DOI: 10.1016/S0140-6736(10)60491-6

[30] Me M, Luna DR, Pagol J, et al. Impact of time to treatment on tissue-type plasminogen activator-induced recanalization in acute ischemic stroke. Stroke. 2014;**45**:2734-2738. DOI: 10.1161/STROKEAHA.114.006222

[31] Campbell BCV, Ma H, Ringleb PA, et al. Extending thrombolysis to 4.5-9 h andwake-up stroke using perfusion imaging: A systematic review and meta-analysis of individual patient data. Lancet. 2019;**394**(10193):139-147. DOI: 10.1016/S0140-6736(19)31053-0

[32] Wahlgren N, Ahmed N, Davalos A, et al. Thrombolysis with alteplase for acute ischaemic stroke in the safe implementation of thrombolysis in stroke-monitoring study (SITS-MOST):

An observational study. Lancet. 2007;**369**:275-282. DOI: 10.1016/ S0140-6736(07)60149-4

[33] Yaghi S, Willey JZ, Cucchiara B, et al. Treatment and outcome of hemorrhagic transformation after intravenous alteplase in acute ischemic stroke a scientific statement for healthcare professionals from the American Heart Association/ American Stroke Association. Stroke. 2017;**48**(12):e343-e361. DOI: 10.1161/ STR.0000000000000152

[34] Myslimi F, Caparros F, Dequatre-Ponchelle N, et al. Orolingual angioedema during or after thrombolysis for cerebral ischemia. Stroke. 2016;**47**:1825-1830. DOI: 10.1161/STROKEAHA.116.013334

[35] Cheong E, Dodd L, Smith W, et al. Icatibant as a potential treatment of life-threatening alteplase-induced angioedema. Journal of Stroke and Cerebrovascular Diseases. 2018; **27**:e36-e37. DOI: 10.1016/j. jstrokecerebrovasdis.2017.09.039

[36] Bivard A, Huang X, Levi CR, et al. Tenecteplase in ischemic strokeoffers improved recanalization: Analysis of 2 trials. Neurology. 2017;**89**:62-67. DOI: 10.1212/WNL.0000000000004062

[37] Campbell BCV, Mitchell PJ, Churilov L, et al. Tenecteplase versus alteplase before thrombectomy for ischemic stroke. The New England Journal of Medicine. 2018;**378**:1573-1582. DOI: 10.1056/NEJMoa1716405

[38] Logallo N, Novotny V, Assmus J, et al. Tenecteplase versus alteplase for management of acute ischaemic stroke (NOR-TEST): A phase 3, randomised, open-label, blinded endpoint trial. Lancet Neurology. 2017;**16**(10):781-788. DOI: 10.1016/S1474-4422(17)30253-3

[39] Campbell BCV, Mitchell PJ, Churilov L, et al. Effect of intravenous tenecteplase dose on cerebral

reperfusion before thrombectomy in patients with large vessel occlusion ischemic stroke: The EXTEND-IA TNK part 2 randomized clinical trial. Journal of the American Medical Association. 2020;**323**:1257-1265. DOI: 10.1001/ jama.2020.1511

[40] Campbell BCV, Khatri P. Stroke. Lancet. 2020;**396**(10244):129-142. DOI: 10.1016/S0140-6736(20)31179-X

[41] Powers WJ, Rabinstein AA, Ackerson T, et al. 2018 guidelines for the early management of patients with acute ischemic stroke: A guideline for healthcare professionals from the American Heart Association/American Stroke Association. Stroke. 2018;**49**(3):e46-e110. DOI: 10.1161/ STR.0000000000000158

[42] Burgos AM, Saver JL. Evidence that tenecteplase is noninferior to alteplase for acute ischemic stroke: Meta-analysis of 5 randomized trials. Stroke. 2019;**50**(8):2156-2162. DOI: 10.1161/ STROKEAHA.119.025080

[43] Hacke W, Kaste M, Fieschi C, et al. Randomised double-blind placebo-controlled trial of thrombolytic therapy with intravenous alteplase in acute ischaemic stroke (ECASS II). Second European-Australasian Acute Stroke Study Investigators Lancet 1998;352: 1245-1251. DOI: 10.1016/s0140-6736(98)08020-9

[44] Clark WM, Wissman S, Albers GW, et al. Recombinant tissue-type plasminogen activator (Alteplase) for ischemic stroke 3 to 5 hours after symptom onset. The ATLANTIS study: A randomized controlled trial. Alteplase thrombolysis for acute noninterventional therapy in ischemic stroke. Journal of the American Medical Association. 1999;**282**:2019-2026. DOI: 10.1001/jama.282.21.2019

[45] Hacke W, Kaste M, Bluhmki E, et al. Thrombolysis with alteplase 3 to 4.5

hours after acute ischemic stroke. The New England Journal of Medicine. 2008;**359**(13):1317-1329. DOI: 10.1056/ NEJMoa0804656

[46] Yamaguchi T, Mori E, Minematsu K, et al. Alteplase at 0.6 mg/kg for acute ischemic stroke within 3 hours of onset: Japan alteplase clinical trial (J-ACT). Stroke. 2006;**37**(7):1810-1815. DOI: 10.1161/01.STR.0000227191. 01792.e3

[47] Toyoda K, Koga M, Naganuma M, et al. Routine use of intravenous low-dose recombinant tissue plasminogen activator in Japanese patients: General outcomes and prognostic factors from the SAMURAI register. Stroke. 2009;**40**(11):3591-3595. DOI: 10.1161/ STROKEAHA.109.562991

[48] Minematsu K, Okada Y, et al. Thrombolysis with 0.6 mg/kg intravenous alteplse for acute ischemic stroke in routine clinical practice: The Japan post-marketing alteplse registration study (J-MARS). Stroke. 2010;**41**(9):1984-1989. DOI: 10.1161/ STROKEAHA.110.589606

[49] Sharma VK, Kawnayn G, Sarkar N. Acute ischemic stroke: Comparison of low-dose and standard-dose regimes of tissue plasminogen activator. Expert Review of Neurotherapeutics. 2013;**13**:895-902. DOI: 10.1586/14737175. 2013.827412

[50] Cheng JW, Zhang XJ, Cheng LS, et al. Low-dose tissue plasminogen activator in acute ischemic stroke: A systematic review and meta-analysis. Journal of Stroke and Cerebrovascular Diseases. 2018;**27**:381-390. DOI: 10.1016/j.jstrokecerebrovasdis

[51] Anderson CS, Robinson T, Lindley RI, et al. Low-dose versus standard-dose intravenous alteplase in acute ischemic stroke. The New England Journal of Medicine. 2016;**374**(24):2313- 2323. DOI: 10.1056/NEJMoa1515510

[52] Zhao G, Huang T, Zheng M, et al. Comparative analysis on low- and standard-dose regimes of alteplase thrombolytic therapy for acute ischemic stroke: Efficacy and safety. European Neurology. 2018;**79**(1-2):68-73. DOI: 10.1159/000485460

[53] Liu H, Zheng H, Cao Y, et al. Low- versus standard-dose intravenous tissue plasminogen activator for acute ischemic stroke: An updated meta-analysis. Journal of Stroke and Cerebrovascular Diseases. 2018;**27**(4):988-997. DOI: 10.1016/j. jstrokecerebrovasdis.2017.11.005

[54] Saver JL, Adeoye O. Intravenous thrombolysis before endovascular thrombectomy for acute ischemic stroke. Journal of the American Medical Association. 2020;**325**(3):229-231. DOI: 10.1001/jama.2020.22388

[55] Chalos V, LeCouffe NE, Uyttenboogaart M, et al. Endovascular treatment with or without prior intravenous alteplase for acute ischemic stroke. Journal of the American Heart Association. 2019;**8**(11):e011592

[56] Vidale S, Romoli M, Consoli D, et al. Bridging versus direct mechanical thrombectomy in acute ischemic stroke: A subgroup pooled meta-analysis for time of intervention, eligibility, and study design. Cerebrovascular Diseases. 2020;**49**:223-232

[57] Young-Saver DF, Gornbein J, Starkman S, et al. Magnitude of benefit of combined endovascular thrombectomy and intravenous fibrinolysis in large vessel occlusion ischemic stroke. Stroke. 2019;**50**: 2433-2440

[58] Yang P, Zhang Y, Zhang L, et al. Endovascular thrombectomy with or without intravenous alteplase in acute stroke. The New England Journal of Medicine. 2020;**382**(21):1981-1993. DOI: 10.1056/NEJMoa2001123

[59] Zi W, Qiu Z, Li F, et al. Effect of endovascular treatment alone vs intravenous alteplase plus endovascular treatment on functional independence in patients with acute ischemic stroke. Journal of the American Medical Association. 2021;**325**(3):234-243. DOI: 10.1001/jama.2020.23523

[60] TC-Sağlık Bakanlığı Sağlık Hizmetleri Genel Müdürlüğü. Akut iskemik inme tanı ve tedavi rehberi. Ankara; 2020. Available from: https://sbu.saglik.gov.tr/Ekutuphane/Yayin/566.

[61] Peter-Derex L, Derex L. Wake-up stroke: From pathophysiology to management. Sleep Medicine Reviews. 2019;**48**:101212. DOI: 10.1016/j.smrv.2019.101212

[62] Wang C, Wang W, Ji J, et al. Safety of intravenous thrombolysis in stroke of unknown time of onset: A systematic review and meta-analysis. Journal of Thrombosis and Thrombolysis. 2021. Online ahead of print. DOI: 10.1007/s11239-021-02476-6

[63] Berge E, Whiteley W, Audebert H, et al. European Stroke Organisation (ESO) guidelines on intravenous thrombolysis for acute ischaemic stroke. European Stroke Journal. 2021;**6**(1):I-LXII. DOI: 10.1177/2396987321989865

[64] Koga M, Yamamoto H, Inoue M, et al. Thrombolysis with alteplase at 0.6 mg/kg for stroke with unknown time of onset: A randomized controlled trial. Stroke. 2020;**51**(5):1530-1538. DOI: 10.1161/STROKEAHA.119.028127

[65] Ringleb P, Bendszus M, Bluhmki E, et al. Extending the time window for intravenous thrombolysis in acute ischemic stroke using magnetic resonance imaging-based patient selection. International Journal of Stroke. 2019;**14**(5):483-490. DOI: 10.1177/1747493019840938

[66] Furlanis G, Ajčević M, Buoite Stella A, et al. Wake-up stroke: Thrombolysis reduces ischemic lesion volume and neurological deficit. Journal of Neurology. 2020;**267**:666-673. DOI: 10.1007/s00415-019-09603-7

[67] Swartz RH, Cayley ML, Foley N. The incidence of pregnancy-related stroke: A systematic review and meta-analysis. International Journal of Stroke. 2017;**12**(7):687-697. DOI: 10.1177/1747493017723271

[68] Khalid AS, Hadbavna A, Williams D, et al. A review of stroke in pregnancy: Incidence, investigations and management. The Obstetrician & Gynaecologist. 2020;**22**:21-33. DOI: 10.1111/tog.12624

[69] Tate J, Bushnell C. Pregnancy and stroke risk in women. Womens Health. 2011;**7**(3):363-374. DOI: 10.2217/whe.11.19

[70] Little JT, Bookwalter CA. Magnetic resonance safety: Pregnancy and lactation. Magnetic Resonance Imaging Clinics of North America. 2020;**28**(4):509-516. DOI: 10.1016/j.mric.2020.06.002

[71] Anderson A, Singh J, Bove R. Neuroimaging and radiation exposure in pregnancy. Handbook of Clinical Neurology. 2020;**171**:179-191. DOI: 10.1016/B978-0-444-64239-4.00009-6

[72] Gartman EJ. The use of thrombolytic therapy in pregnancy. Obstetric Medicine. 2013;**6**(3):105-111. DOI: 10.1177/1753495X13488771

[73] Landais A, Chaumont H, Dellis R. Thrombolytic therapy of acute ischemic stroke during early pregnancy. Journal of Stroke and Cerebrovascular Diseases. 2018;**27**(2):e20-e23. DOI: 10.1016/j.jstrokecerebrovasdis

[74] Rodrigues R, Silva R, Fontão L. Acute ischemic stroke in pregnancy. Case Reports in Neurology. 2019;**11**(1):37-40. DOI: 10.1159/000496386

[75] Dinehart E, Leon Guerrero C, Pham A. Extending the window for thrombolysis for treatment of acute ischaemic stroke during pregnancy: A review. BJOG : An International Journal of Obstetrics and Gynaecology. 2021;**128**:516-520. DOI: 10.1111/ 1471-0528.16495

[76] Pacheco LD, Hankins GDV, Saad AF. Acute management of ischemic stroke during pregnancy. Obstetrics and Gynecology. 2019;**133**(5):933-939. DOI: 10.1097/AOG.0000000000003220

[77] Keselman B, Gdovinová Z, Jatuzis D. Safety and outcomes of intravenous thrombolysis in posterior versus anterior circulation stroke: Results from the safe implementation of treatments in stroke registry and meta-analysis. Stroke. 2020;**51**(3):876-882. DOI: 10.1161/STROKEAHA. 119.027071

[78] Dorňák T, Sedláčková Z, Čivrný J, et al. Brain imaging findings and response to intravenous thrombolysis in posterior circulation stroke. Advances in Therapy. 2021;**38**(1):627-639. DOI: 10.1007/ s12325-020-01547-z

[79] Rabinstein AA. Treatment of acute ischemic stroke. Cerebrovascular Disease. 2017;**23**:62-81. DOI: 10.1212/ CON.0000000000000420

[80] Pallesen LP, Khomenko A, Dzialowski I, et al. CT-angiography source images indicate less fatal outcome despite coma of patients in the Basilar Artery International Cooperation Study. International Journal of Stroke. 2017;**2**:145-151. DOI: 10.1177/1747493016669886

[81] Dornak T, Kral M, Sanak D, et al. Intravenos thrombolysis in posterior circulation stroke. Frontiers in Neurology. 2019;**10**:417. DOI: 10.3389/ fneur.2019.00417

Chapter 8

Infarct Stroke and Blood Glucose Associated with Food Consumption in Indonesia

Santi Martini, Hermina Novida and Kuntoro

Abstract

Stroke is the primary cause of death in adults. It is predicted that the death caused by stroke will increase twice in the next 30 years. In Indonesia, stroke is one of the diseases of the circulatory system, which has been taking the first place of causing death since 2007. Indonesia has rice as the main type of daily food consumed, which has higher glycemic index than other sources. This study aims to find the risk of blood glucose level that determines the incidence of infarct stroke. There were 164 patients enrolled in this study, 82 patients in each stroke and not stroke group. The blood examination is using the enzymatic method, which is the hexokinase method. The results of research revealed that indicators of high blood glucose level were found in infract stroke incidence, including casual blood glucose, fasting blood glucose, 2-h postprandial blood glucose, and glycated hemoglobin. These four indicators were found in a higher level in the infarct stroke than the non-stroke group. Other epidemiological studies have shown that diabetes is a risk factor for stroke. Therefore, education about food selection should be a priority in the effort to prevent infarct stroke and diabetes mellitus in Indonesia.

Keywords: infarct stroke, cerebrovascular disease, blood glucose, diabetes, tobacco use, Indonesia

1. Introduction

Stroke was previously assumed to occur in developed countries only, as the third leading cause of death and is responsible for 5.5 million deaths every year [1, 2]. However, it is actually uncommon to be found in Southeast Asian countries [3–5] or other countries with low and middle income [6].

Stroke is the primary cause of death and disability in the world, whose cost needed for post-stroke treatment and care is quite pricey. In 2016, stroke was the second leading cause of death globally (5.5 million deaths) after ischemic heart disease [2]. In South Asian countries including India, Pakistan, and Bangladesh, as well as developing countries in Southeast Asia, such as Cambodia, Indonesia, Laos, and Malaysia, the stroke incidence is increasing. However, since these developing countries do not have inadequate health facilities, the mortality rate caused by this disease is high and the number of persons with disabilities caused by this disease also increases [3, 7–9].

Stroke is the leading cause of death in adults. The death caused by stroke is predicted to increase twice in the next 30 years [10]. A previous research project carried out by

Carandang (2006) discovered that approximately 62% of all stroke cases were athero-thrombotic infarcts [11]. Meanwhile, according to Puthenpurakal [12] about 85% of stroke cases are ischemic stroke or infarct stroke, while the remaining (15%) are hemorrhagic stroke. Global data issued in 2016 also gave similar results, in which 84.4% of stroke incidence were ischemic stroke [2]. Stroke with ischemic health diseases (IHD) was the leading cause of deaths attributable to tobacco use as a risk factor [13].

According to Basic Health Research (RISKESDAS) that was conducted in Indonesia in 2007, it was revealed that stroke was the leading cause of death by 15.4% [14]. In the age group of 45 to 54 years old, stroke is the leading cause of death in urban areas and in men. Meanwhile, in the age group of 55 to 64 years old, this disease is the leading cause of death in both urban and rural areas as well as in both male and female [14]. Martini et al. [15] revealed that 76% of stroke incidence in a hospital that has been a tertiary referral in the last 10 years was ischemic stroke or infarct stroke. Furthermore, there was also an increase of stroke incidence in 2013 compared to 2007, which was 12.1 and 8.3% [14, 16]. Meanwhile, the stroke incidence in 2018 was 10.9 per mile [17].

Previous study carried out by Pinto et al. showed that hypertension was commonly found in lacunar infarct stroke and large artery atherosclerosis in diabetic patients [18]. Therefore, it indicates that hypertension is a co-factor that determines lacunar stroke in diabetic patients. This is in accordance with the statement made by Harry Keen three decades ago that both high blood glucose level and high blood pressure damage blood vessels, especially the small blood vessels (microvascular). Meanwhile, research conducted by Kisella et al. [19] claimed that hypertension comorbidity was not a significant risk factor for the stroke infarct incidence in African Americans (OR = 1.3 95% confidence interval [CI]: 0.9–1.7), yet it was a significant risk factor for the infarct stroke incidence in Caucasian people (OR = 1.6, 95% CI: 1.4–1.9). About 35–42% of all infarct stroke incidences in both African Americans and Caucasians are related to diabetes alone or in combination between diabetes and hypertension. The risk of stroke in hypertension was 1.46 (95% CI: 1.07–1.99) as the sole risk factor [20]. Hypertension is the most common risk factor found in Asia 1 [3, 4, 21, 22]. Data from one of the community-based surveys in Indonesia, which is Sleman Health and Demographic Surveillance System (HDSS) in 2016, found a high prevalence of stroke that was related to the increasing age, hypertension, and diabetes mellitus [9].

When diabetes mellitus (DM) is the sole factor, then DM also increases the risk of infarct stroke [23, 24]. Furthermore, the risk of infarct stroke is 2.5 (95% CI: 2.0–3.2) in all types of DM. According to the type of diabetes mellitus, the risk of infarct stroke is 7.9 times (95% CI: 5.1–12.2) in DM type 1 and 3.0 times (95% CI: 2.6–3.4) in DM type 2. Meanwhile, based on the duration of suffering from DM type 2, infarct stroke risk increases by 1.7 times when the duration of illness is less than 5 years and 3.2 times when the duration of illness is within 10–14 years [25]. Diabetes patients have a higher risk ([OR] 1.33, 95% CI: 1.18–1.5) of suffering from ischemic stroke than hemorrhagic stroke (OR 0.72, 95% CI: 0.6–0.877). In addition, the combination of infarct stroke and DM affects younger people more than infarct stroke without DM. The risk of infarct stroke is more common in white DM patients [26]. According to research conducted by Kaarisalo et al. [27], infarct stroke has a tendency to occur more frequently in people with impaired glucose tolerance (GTG) than in people with normal blood glucose levels, although the difference was not significant [28]. In addition, several studies have estimated that approximately 20–33% of hospitalized patients with acute stroke have diabetes [29, 30]. This is strengthened by the results of the research conducted at General Hospital of Haji Adam Malik Medan Indonesia that diabetes had a relationship with the prevalence of stroke ($p < 0.05$). The risk of stroke was 1.34 times higher in diabetes than those without diabetes [30].

Stroke can occur in all age groups but mostly occurs at the age above 55 years old; thus, age is a strong determinant of infarct stroke incidence [9, 31–33]. Many factors cause stroke. An individual may have more than one risk factor, whether the risk factor is a risk factor that is supported by strong evidence (level of evidence A) or less strong evidence (level of evidence C), or whether these risk factors can be modified or cannot be modified, or whether these risk factors are controlled or not.

High blood glucose level can cause complications on blood vessels such as microangiopathy (eye, kidney, and nerve disorders) and macroangiopathy (stroke and heart problems). If the blood glucose is excessive, then glucose will bind to proteins, including blood vessel wall cells. These bonds will damage the structure and function of blood vessels. The damage or complications that occur cannot be reversed and the process can only be stopped or slowed down [34]. Furthermore, hyperglycemia increases oxidative stress, which causes pathological processes in diabetic complications. Overproduction of reactive oxygen species (ROS) induced by hyperglycemia will activate five pathogenic pathways that contribute to endo-thelial dysfunction and diabetes complications, and those are (1) polyol pathway; (2) the increase of formation of advanced glycation end products (AGEs); (3) the increase of receptor expression for AGEs; (4) activation of protein kinase C iso-forms; and (5) over-activity of the hexamine pathway. Vasculopathy that is induced by chronic hyperglycemia also results in accelerated atherosclerosis in diabetes. Therefore, a higher prevalence and incidence of cardiovascular disease including stroke are common in the diabetic patients [35, 36]. Improper diabetes control also increases the short- and long-term morbidity and mortality associated with stroke and significantly increases the recurrent risk of stroke [35].

Based on the doctor diagnosis, the prevalence of diabetes in Indonesia popula-tion has increased from 2007 to 2018. This can be seen from the results of Basic Health Research (RISKESDAS) [16], which increased from 1.5% in 2007 to 2.0% in 2018. Such condition shows that serious problems still occur related to unresolved diabetes. Meanwhile, the prevalence based on the age increased from 2007 to 2018. In this case, the age category was divided into seven groups and the highest preva-lence was shown by the age group of above 55 years old and this figure was related to insulin resistance.

Age is a risk factor for diabetes [37]. Based on the results of the research afore-said, the older age group suffers from DM more. The increasing prevalence of DM that includes metabolic diseases at the old age can be directly related to the aging process or indirectly through several other DM risk factors such as central obesity, mitochondrial dysfunction, FFA and lipid metabolism disorders, inflammation, cell dysfunction, insulin resistance, and metabolic syndrome (**Figure 1**) [38]. The purpose of this study is to find the factor that increases the risk of infarct stroke related to the blood glucose level of Indonesian people.

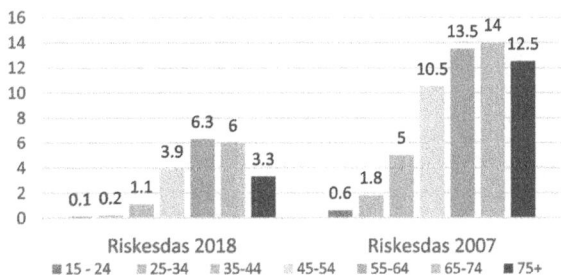

Figure 1.
Prevalence of diabetes mellitus among people age 15 years old and over in Indonesia.

2. Food consumption in Indonesia

Indonesia is the third largest sugar consumer in Asia after India and China. Indonesian people consumption of sugar is slightly higher (5%) than the total energy and when combined with the sugar contained in beverages such as soft drinks, the content will be even higher [39].

Basic Health Research (RISKESDAS) that was conducted in 2018 showed that there were 40.1 and 60.27% of Indonesian people at the age of above 3 years old who consumed sweet foods and beverages once a day [40]. Meanwhile, previous research in 2007 and 2013 found that the consumption of sweet foods was still quite high, although it decreased from 65.2 to 53.1%.

In this case, children at the age group of 3–9 years old have the highest percentage (above 50%) of consuming sweet foods once a day. Furthermore, about 98.4% of Indonesian teenagers at the age of 13–18 years old consumed nutritious foods including fruits and vegetables insufficiently (<400 g/day) [41]. The prevalence of overweight in Indonesia is the highest among adults by 8% of men and 29% of women suffering from central obesity [42]. Therefore, concern needs to be provided to the quality of community diet needs and energy adequacy, especially among teenagers and children who need nutritional intake in the growth process.

Basic Health Research (RISKESDAS) in 2007, 2013, and 2018 was conducted concerning the food consumption pattern of Indonesian people as presented in **Figure 2**. The prevalence of sweet foods and drinks consumption once a day was 65.2% in 2007, which then decreased to 53.1% in 2013. Furthermore, the consumption of sweet food for once a day also decreased to 40.1% in 2018, yet the consumption of sweet beverages once a day increased to 61.27%. In addition, the consumption of soft drinks or carbonated drinks was 2.2% (**Figure 3**) [14, 16, 17, 40].

Several other studies have also revealed that Indonesian adults insufficiently consumed protein, fruits, and vegetables, but consumed fast food and sodium excessively [41]. Another study that has been conducted in Central Java, Indonesia, also showed that dietary patterns were associated with increased consumption of soft drinks, snacks, and various animal products [43]. Another study was further conducted in Jakarta showing that the daily food consumption of the observed population reached 1868–2334 g/capita/day. The total intake of added sugar in the different groups of respondents ranged between 34.9 and 45.9 g/capita/day, with the highest values observed in school-age boys. Total salt intake ranged from 5.46 to 7.43 g/capita/day, while fat intake reached 49.0–65.1 g/capita/day. One of the main food sources that contribute to salt and fat intake is street food and fast-food restaurants [44].

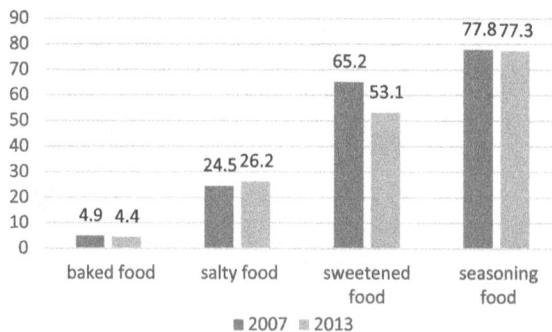

Figure 2.
The percentage of population aged 10 years and older to consume unhealthy food ≥1 per day in Indonesia in 2007 and 2013.

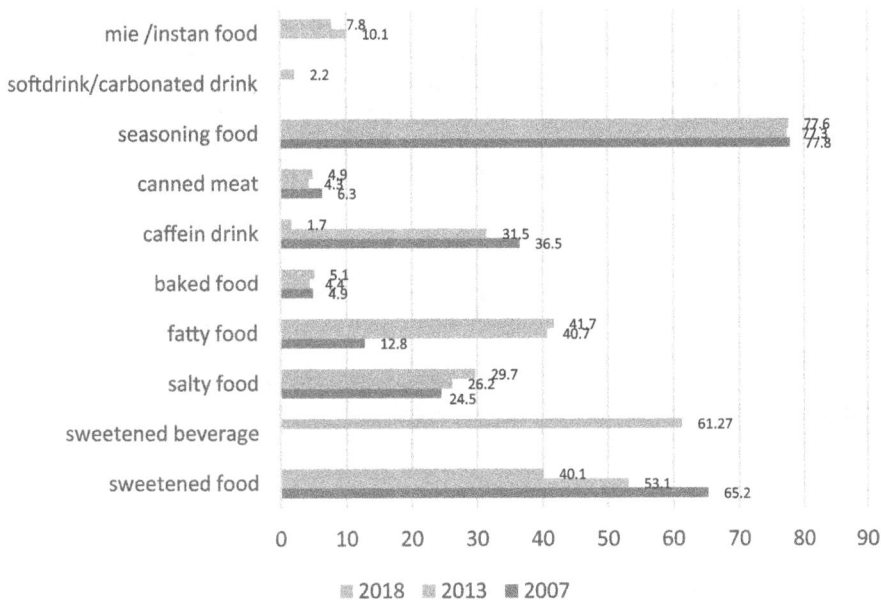

Figure 3.
Unhealthy food consumption based on Basic Health Research (RISKESDAS) 2007, 2013, and 2018.

3. Data and analysis

The population involved is those who suffered from infarct stroke and were treated at RSUD Dr. Soetomo. The population source was hospital-based because, to obtain data on stroke incidence, it must be based on a doctor's diagnosis, not based on the results of interviews. Case samples were infarct stroke incidences, which were taken by consecutive sampling from the case population with several inclusion criteria, including (1) aged 40 years and above, (2) male and female, (3) normal consciousness (GCS 4 5 6), and (4) willing to participate in the research (proven by informed consent). Meanwhile, the exclusion criteria were (1) having family comorbidity of stroke, (2) previous heart disease (proven by being hospitalized with a diagnosis of heart disease), and (3) aphasia. Furthermore, the sampling was carried out in the Neurology Inpatient Ward of RSUD Dr. Soetomo in Surabaya, Indonesia.

Based on the calculation, there were 79 samples obtained from each group. In this research, there were 82 samples for each group; thus, there were 164 samples involved. Data collection was carried out through several stages. The first stage is conducting direct examination of research subjects to obtain a diagnosis of infarct stroke (based on clinical signs, symptoms, and CT scan images) when the respondent arrived at the hospital. Second stage is examining the blood sugar, by collecting venous blood through taking 3 µl of serum added by 200 µl of reagent 1 and 200 µl of reagent 2, then incubated for 10 minutes, and read at wavelengths of 600 and 505 nm. The examination method used is the enzymatic method, which is the hexokinase method. This method was chosen because it has good precision and accuracy and is a referential method [45]. Casual blood sugar and HBA_{1C} examinations were carried out no later than 24 h after the respondents entered the nervous room [46]. After that, the respondents were required to fast for at least 10 h to check the fasting blood sugar in the next day. Then, respondents were asked to eat rice (the menu provided by the hospital) and 2 h after eating, and their blood was taken for blood sugar examination 2-h postprandial for cases. During the controls, casual blood sugar and HBA$_{1C}$ tests were carried out before the interview, and then, respondents were asked to fast for at least 10 h before having their blood drawn the next day for fasting blood sugar checks. After the blood was taken, respondents were asked to eat rice, side dishes, and drink sweet tea equivalent to 600 to 650 calories. The respondents' blood was then taken again 2 h after eating for blood sugar examination 2-h postprandial. The examination results were categorized according to the *American Diabetes Association* (ADA) criteria and percentiles based on the average of these examination results.

This research employed a research instrument in the form of a questionnaire to obtain data on age, gender, blood sugar, medical history, which is diabetes mellitus. A computerized (CT) scan of the head was further conducted as the gold standard to determine the diagnosis of infarct stroke and to check serum sugar and cholesterol levels using the Hitachi 912 autoanalyzer.

4. Results and discussion

4.1 Results

4.1.1 Casual blood glucose according to infarct stroke status

The results showed that the average casual blood glucose (CBG) was 148.57 mg/dl with the lowest CBG level was 66 mg/dl and the highest CBG was 535 mg/dl. Based on the Kolmogorov–Smirnov normality test, p-value obtained was 0.000 indicating that the distribution of CBG data did not show a normal distribution. Therefore, CBG was classified according to the percentile method as follows:

Group I: CBG < 87 mg/dl
Group II: CBG 87 to 224 mg/dl
Group III: CBG > 224 mg/dl

The mean value of CBG in the infarct stroke was 186 mg/dl with a standard deviation of 14 mg/dl. Meanwhile, the mean value of CBG in the non-stroke group was 111 mg/dl with a standard deviation of 65 mg/dl.

This casual blood glucose (CBG) was categorized based on the *American Diabetes Association* (ADA) 2010 criteria [46]. The percentile method is shown in **Table 1**. Based on **Table 1**, there were only 4.9% of respondents who had CBG of 87 mg/dl in the infarct stroke group. Meanwhile, in the non-stroke group, almost 30% of respondents had CBG of 87 mg/dl. Furthermore, according to the criteria of percentile method, there were 28% of respondents who had CBG 224 mg/dl in the infarct stroke group and 4.9% of respondents with CBG 224 mg/dl in the non-stroke group. Furthermore, according to the ADA criteria, almost 50% of infarct stroke incidence had CBG levels of 140 mg/dl and above. On the other hand, 90.3% of non-stroke incidences had CBG level of less than 140 mg/dl.

4.1.2 Fasting blood glucose based on infarct stroke status

Fasting blood glucose (FBG) was categorized based on *American Diabetes Association* (ADA) 2010 criteria and percentile method as presented in **Table 2**. The fasting blood glucose (FBG) variable had an average fasting blood glucose level (FBG) of 114.07 mg/dl with the lowest fasting blood glucose level was 65 mm Hg, while the highest fasting blood glucose was 329 mg/dl. Based on the Kolmogorov–Smirnov normality test, the p-value obtained was 0.000, indicating that the

Disease	Casual blood glucose	Number	Percentage
Infarct stroke			
ADA criteria	<140 mg/dl	42	51.2
	140–199 mg/dl	13	15.9
	> = 200 mg/dl	27	32.9
Percentile method	<87 mg/dl	4	4.9
	87–224 mg/dl	55	67.1
	>224 mg/dl	23	28.0
Not stroke			
ADA criteria	<140 mg/dl	74	90.3
	140–199 mg/dl	2	2.4
	> = 200 mg/dl	6	7.3
Percentile method	<87 mg/dl	24	29.3
	87–224 mg/dl	54	65.9
	>224 mg/dl	4	4.9

Table 1.
Distribution of casual blood glucose (CBG) of the respondents based on the infarct stroke status according to the American Diabetes Association (ADA) 2010 criteria and percentile method.

Disease	Fasting blood glucose	Number	Percentage
Infarct stroke			
ADA criteria	<110 mg/dl	37	45.1
	110–125 mg/dl	12	14.6
	> = 126 mg/dl	33	40.2
Percentile method	<80 mg/dl	4	4.9
	80–159 mg/dl	54	65.9
	>159 mg/dl	24	29.3
Not stroke			
ADA criteria	<110 mg/dl	71	86.6
	110–125 mg/dl	5	6.1
	> = 126 mg/dl	6	7.3
Percentile method	<80 mg/dl	19	23.2
	80–159 mg/dl	61	74.4
	>159 mg/dl	2	2.4

Table 2.
Fasting blood glucose (FBG) of the respondents based on the infarct stroke status according to the American Diabetes Association (ADA) 2010 criteria and percentile method.

distribution of GDP data did not show a normal distribution. Therefore, FBG was classified according to the percentile method as follows:

Groups I: FBG < 80 mg/dl
Groups II: FBG 80 to 159 mg/dl
Groups III: FBG > 159 mg/dl

The average fasting blood glucose (FBG) in the infarct stroke group was 134 mg/dl with a standard deviation of 54 mg/dl, while in the non-stroke group it was 94 mg/dl with a standard deviation of 33 mg/dl.

According to ADA 2010 criteria, in the stroke-infarction group, there were 40.2% of respondents had a FBG level of 126 mg/dl or more, 14.6% of respondents had a FBG of 110 to 125 mg/dl, and 45.1% of respondents had a FBG 110 mg/dl. Meanwhile, in the non-stroke group, most respondents (86.6%) had a FBG of 110 mg/dl and only 7.3% of respondents had a FBG of 126 mg/dl or more. Furthermore, according to the percentile method, in terms of the infarct group, 29.3% of respondents had a FBG level of 159 mg/dl and only 4.9% of respondents had a FBG level of 80 mg/dl, while the remaining (65.9%) had a FBG level of 80 to 159 mg/dl. Meanwhile, in the non-stroke group, as many as 23.2% of respondents had a FBG of 80 mg/dl, only 2.4% had a FBG of more than 159 mg/dl, and 74.4% of the respondents had a FBG of 80 to 159 mg/dl.

4.1.3 Blood glucose of 2-h postprandial according to the infarct stroke status

The mean value of blood glucose of 2-h postprandial (BG2PP) was 144.32 mg/dl with the lowest blood glucose levels of 2-h postprandial was 68 mg/dl, while the highest was 483 mg/dl. Based on the Kolmogorov–Smirnov normality test, the p-value obtained was 0.000 indicating that the distribution of BG2PP data did not show a normal distribution. Therefore, BG2PP was classified according to the percentile method as follows:

Group I: BG2PP < 94 mg/dl
Group II: BG2PP 94 to 207 mg/dl
Group III: BG2PP > 207 mg/dl

The mean blood glucose of 2-h postprandial (BG2PP) in the infarct stroke group was 165 mg/dl with a standard deviation of 70 mg/dl, while in the non-stroke group was 124 mg/dl with a standard deviation of 62 mg/dl.

The blood glucose of 2-h postprandial (BG2PP) was categorized based on the American Diabetes Association (ADA) criteria 2010 and the percentile method as presented in **Table 3**.

According to the ADA criteria 2010, in terms of infarct stroke, there were 28% of respondents who had a BG2PP level of 200 mg/dl or more, 18.3% of respondents had a BG2PP level of 140 to 200 mg/dl, and 53.7% of respondents had a BG2PP level of 140 mg/dl. On the other hand, in terms of the non-stroke group, most of the respondents (84.1%) had a BG2PP level of 140 mg/dl and only 7.3% of respondents had a BG2PP level of 200 mg/dl or more. Meanwhile, according to the percentile method in the stroke-infarction group, there were 62.2% of respondents which

Disease	Blood glucose of 2 hours post-prandial	Number	Percentage
Infarct stroke			
ADA criteria	<140 mg/dl	44	53.7
	140–199 mg/dl	15	18.3
	> = 200 mg/dl	23	28.0
Percentile method	<94 mg/dl	11	13.4
	94–207 mg/dl	51	62.2
	>207 mg/dl	20	24.4
Not stroke			
ADA criteria	<140 mg/dl	69	84.1
	140–199 mg/dl	7	8.5
	> = 200 mg/dl	6	7.3
Percentile method	<94 mg/dl	21	25.6
	94–207 mg/dl	55	67.1
	>207 mg/dl	6	7.3

Table 3.
Blood glucose of 2 hours post-prandial (BG2PP) of the respondents based on the infarct stroke status according to the American Diabetes Association (ADA) 2010 criteria and percentile method.

had a BG2PP level of 94–207 mg/dl and 24.4% of respondents with BG2PP level of 207 mg/dl. Meanwhile, in the non-stroke group, there were 25.6% of respondents, which had a BG2PP level of 94 mg/dl, 67.1% of respondents had 94 to 207 mg/dl, and only 7.3% of respondents had a BG2PP level of more than 207 mg/dl.

4.1.4 Hemoglobin glycated (HBA$_{1c}$) according to the infarct stroke status

Variable of glycated hemoglobin (HBA$_{1C}$) level obtained the mean value of 6.37%. The lowest HBA$_{1C}$ level was 3.5%, while the highest was 11.6%. Based on the Kolmogorov–Smirnov normality test, the p = value obtained was 0.011, indicating that the HBA$_{1C}$ data distribution did not show a normal distribution. Therefore, HBA$_{1C}$ was classified according to the percentile method as follows:

Group I: HBA$_{1C}$ < 6.1%

Group II: HBA$_{1C}$ ≥ 6.1%

The mean value of HBA$_{1C}$ level in the stroke infarct group was 7.07% with a standard deviation of 1.40%. Meanwhile, the mean value in the non-stroke group was 5.74% with a standard deviation of 0.97%. Furthermore, the HBA$_{1C}$ levels were categorized according to the American Diabetes Association (ADA) criteria 2010 and the percentile method as described in **Table 4**.

According to the ADA criteria 2010, in the infarct stroke group, there were 67.1% of respondents who had HBA$_{1C}$ level of 6% or more, while the remaining obtained HBA$_{1C}$ level less than 6%. On the other hand, in the non-stroke group, most (64.6%) of the respondents obtained HBA$_{1C}$ level of less than 6%, while 35.4% respondents had HBA$_{1C}$ level of 6% or more.

According to the percentile method, in the infarct stroke group, there were 63.4% of respondents who had HBA$_{1C}$ level of 6.1% or more, while the remaining 36.6% of respondents had HBA$_{1C}$ level of less than 6.1%. On the other hand, in the non-stroke group, there were 67.1% of respondents who had HBA$_{1C}$ level of less than 6.1%, while the remaining 32.9% of respondents had HBA$_{1C}$ level of 6.1% or more.

4.2 Discussion

Based on the results that have been described above, it was discovered that the variable of blood glucose in the stroke infarct group was higher than the non-stroke group's. The mean value of casual blood glucose (CBG) in the infarct stroke group

Disease	HBA$_{1C}$ level	Number	Percentage
Infarct stroke			
ADA criteria	< 6.0%	27	32.9
	> = 6.0%	55	67.1
Percentile method	< 6.1%	30	36.6
	> = 6.1%	52	63.4
Not Stroke			
ADA criteria	< 6.0%	53	64.6
	> = 6.0%	29	35.4
Percentile method	< 6.1%	55	67.1
	> = 6.1%	27	32.9

Table 4.
Hemoglobin glycated (HBA$_{1C}$) level of the respondents based on the infarct stroke status according to the American Diabetes Association (ADA) 2010 criteria and percentile method.

was 186 mg/dl, while the mean value of CBG in the non-stroke group was 111 mg/dl. Meanwhile, the fasting blood glucose (FBG) level in the infarct stroke group was 134 mg/dl, while in the non-stroke group it was 94 mg/dl. Furthermore, the blood sugar of 2-h postprandial (BG2PP) in the infarct stroke group was 165 mg/dl, while in the non-stroke group it was 124 mg/dl. These results supported the results of previous research conducted by Berger et al. [47] in which the FBG level in the stroke group was higher than in the non-stroke group, which was 106.1 mg/dl and 101.1 mg/dl, respectively.

Furthermore, another previous research project carried out by Boden-Albala et al. [48] revealed that the increase of FBG levels caused the risk of ischemic stroke also increased by 2.7 (95% CI: 2.0–3.8). In addition, it was reported that FBG level of 126 mg/dl to less than 150 mg/dl had a 5.1 (95%CI: 2.8–9.3) risk of ischemic stroke, while if the FBG level is 150 mg/dl, it had a risk of 3.3 (95%CI: 2.2–4.8).

Blood glucose level examination is an examination carried out to determine a definite diagnosis of diabetes mellitus. If the American Diabetes Association (ADA) 2010 criteria were used to determine the diagnosis of diabetes mellitus, the blood sugar level of 2-h post-prandial obtained that 28% of respondents have diabetes mellitus. This percentage figure is higher than the figure obtained from the research performed by O'Donnel et al. [49], in which 21% of ischemic stroke cases had diabetes mellitus. The results of this study are in accordance with previous studies that diabetes mellitus is a factor that increases the risk of ischemic stroke with a risk of 2.2 (95% CI: 1.9–2.6) [28] and a high risk of 1.78 (95% CI: 1.32–2.42) [50] while based on the gender, it was 2.27 (95% CI: 2.24–2.29) for men and 2.15 (95% CI: 2.13–2.17) for women [50, 51].

Other epidemiological studies have shown that diabetes is a risk factor for either ischemic stroke or infarct stroke or hemorrhagic stroke [30]. For example, findings from the Emerging Risk Factors Collaboration showed that the hazard ratio (HR) with diabetes was 2.27 (95% CI: 1.95–2.65) for ischemic stroke or infarct stroke, 1.56 (95% CI: 1.19–2.05) for hemorrhagic stroke, and 1.84 (95% CI: 1.59–2.13) for unclassified stroke [28, 52]. A cohort study was conducted in Taiwan, obtaining that the stroke incidence with and without diabetes was 10.1 and 4.5 per 1000 person-year, respectively. During the follow-up, diabetic patients had an increased risk of stroke (adjusted hazard ratio 1.75; 95%CI: 1.64–1.86) than those without diabetes. The relationship between diabetes and stroke risk was significant in both genders and all age groups [22].

In the glycated hemoglobin variable (HBA_{1C}), the average HBA_{1C} in the infarct stroke group was higher than the non-stroke group, which was 7.07 and 5.74%, respectively. Elevated glycated hemoglobin (HBA_{1C}) was an independent predictor of cardiovascular disease with a risk of 1.06 (95%CI: 1.02–1.11) [53]. In addition, the high HBA_{1C} level (>10.7%) was strongly related to stroke [47]. Diabetes is the most important risk factor for ischemic stroke either with diabetes mellitus alone or in combination between diabetes mellitus and hypertension [22, 29, 54]. Another study showed that the ischemic stroke group had significantly higher HBA_{1C} levels (5.9 ± 2.9% vs. 5.5 ± 1.6%) compared with the control group, while HBA_{1C} was a significant determinant of stroke ($p < 0.05$). HBA_{1C} was also significantly higher in the diabetic group compared with the non-diabetic (7.6 ± 2.1 vs. 6.1 ± 2.3) ($p < 0.05$) (7.6 ± 2.1 vs. 6.1 ± 2.3) ($p < 0.05$) [55].

In the current research, the blood glucose variable is a variable, which is strongly related to the incidence of infarct stroke because the highest consumption of carbohydrates in Indonesia is rice (1433 kcal/person/day), corn (228 kcal/person/day), and cassava (161 kcal/person/day) based on data from FAO. Based on the glycemic index, rice and corn have a high glycemic index (GI), which is more than 85 [56].

Variable	Validity		Reliability	
	coefficient	*p-value*	coefficient	*p-value*
Cigarette smoke exposure	0.16	0.05	0.97	0.00
History of hypertension	0.27	0.00	0.93	0.00
History of diabetes	0.73	0.00	0.46	0.00
History of hiperurisemia	0.17	0.00	0.97	0.00
Systolic blood pressure	0.50	0.00	0.75	0.00
Diastolic blood pressure	0.46	0.00	0.79	0.00
Casual blood glucose	0.93	0.00	0.13	0.00
Fasting blood glucose	0.97	0.00	0.05	0.00
Two hours post-prandial blood glucose	0.93	0.00	0.14	0.00
HBA_{1C}	0.70	0.00	0.52	0.00
Total cholesterol	0.20	0.02	0.96	0.00
HDL cholesterol	0.17	0.04	0.97	0.00

Table 5.
The coefficient of validity (λ), reliability (δ) and t-value of each variable compromising the infarct stroke risk index (IRSI) of type a on the final stage of confirmatory factor analysis.

This causes a large glucose load on the body causing a relative insulin deficiency. As a result, not all glucose can be converted into glycogen, resulting in excessive glucose in the blood, causing hyperglycemia.

Blood glucose level is a valid indicator of the risk of infarct stroke. This is proven when blood sugar variable consisting of casual blood sugar, fasting blood sugar, blood sugar of 2-h postprandial, and HBA_{1C} were analyzed together with the other variables (multivariable analysis). It was revealed that the four variables of blood sugar level showed the greatest validity coefficients based on confirmatory factor analysis, as shown in **Table 5**.

5. Conclusion

In Indonesia, it was revealed that stroke was the leading cause of death by 15.4% in 2007. A study conducted in the tertiary hospital revealed that 76% of stroke incidence in the last 10 years was ischemic stroke or infarct stroke. Another study showed that high prevalence of stroke was related to the increasing age, hypertension, and diabetes mellitus. The risk of stroke was 1.34 times higher in diabetes than those without diabetes.

In the current research, the blood glucose variable is a variable that is strongly related to the incidence of infarct stroke associated with the highest consumption of carbohydrates such as rice that is consumed three times a day in Indonesia, whereas it has a high glycemic index compared with other carbohydrate sources, as well, due to the lifestyle of the Indonesian people who like to eat sweet foods and drink sweet beverages. Therefore, education about food selection should be a priority in the effort to prevent infarct stroke and diabetes mellitus in Indonesia.

Efforts to prevent diabetes mellitus and infarct stroke should be considered since there is an emergence of COVID-19 disease, which has a worsening course and high fatality rate in people with comorbidities such as diabetes mellitus and stroke.

Acknowledgements

The author (Santi Martini) is thankful to author's supervisor when taking doctoral program, and Prof. Dr. Moh. Hasan Machfud (neurolog) and Prof. Dr. Joewono Soeroso (internist) for giving knowledge about stroke and the risk factors.

Conflict of interest

The authors declare no conflict of interest.

Author details

Santi Martini[1*], Hermina Novida[2] and Kuntoro[3]

1 Division of Epidemiology, Faculty of Public Health, Universitas Airlangga, Surabaya, Indonesia

2 Department of Internal, Medicine Faculty of Medicine, Universitas Airlangga, Surabaya, Indonesia

3 Division of Biostatistics, Faculty of Public Health, Universitas Airlangga, Surabaya, Indonesia

*Address all correspondence to: santi-m@fkm.unair.ac.id

IntechOpen

References

[1] Gorelick PB. The global burden of stroke: Persistent and disabling. Lancet Neurology. 2019;**18**(5):417-418. DOI: 10.1016/S1474-4422(19)30030-4

[2] Johnson CO et al. Global, regional, and national burden of stroke, 1990-2016: A systematic analysis for the Global Burden of Disease Study 2016. Lancet Neurology. 2019;**18**(5):439-458. DOI: 10.1016/S1474-4422(19)30034-1

[3] Venketasubramanian N, Yoon BW, Pandian J, Navarro JC. Stroke epidemiology in south, east, and south-east asia: A review. Journal of Stroke. 2017;**19**(3):286-294. DOI: 10.5853/jos.2017.00234

[4] Turana Y et al. Hypertension and stroke in Asia: A comprehensive review from HOPE Asia. Journal of Clinical Hypertension. 2021;**23**(3):513-521. DOI: 10.1111/jch.14099

[5] Zhao D. Epidemiological features of cardiovascular disease in Asia. JACC Asia. 2021;**1**(1):1-13. DOI: 10.1016/j.jacasi.2021.04.007

[6] Pandian JD, Kalkonde Y, Sebastian IA, Felix C, Urimubenshi G, Bosch J. Stroke systems of care in low-income and middle-income countries: Challenges and opportunities. Lancet. 2020;**396**(10260):1443-1451. DOI: 10.1016/S0140-6736(20)31374-X

[7] Kusuma Y, Venketasubramanian N, Kiemas LS, Misbach J. Burden of stroke in Indonesia. International Journal of Stroke. 2009;**4**(5):379-380. DOI: 10.1111/j.1747-4949.2009.00326.x

[8] Mehndiratta MM, Khan M, Mehndiratta P, Wasay M. Stroke in Asia: Geographical variations and temporal trends. Journal of Neurology, Neurosurgery, and Psychiatry. 2014;**85**(12):1308-1312. DOI: 10.1136/jnnp-2013-306992

[9] Setyopranoto I et al. Prevalence of stroke and associated risk factors in sleman district of Yogyakarta Special Region, Indonesia. Stroke Research and Treatment. 2019;**2019**:1-8. DOI: 10.1155/2019/2642458

[10] Elkins JS, Johnston SC. Thirty-year projections for deaths from lschemic ischemic stroke in the United States. Stroke. 2003;**34**(9):2109-2112. DOI: 10.1161/01.STR.0000085829.60324.DE

[11] Jeffrey, S. 2006. Stroke Incidence Down, But Severity Unchanged Over Past 50 Years. http://www.medscape.com/viewarticle/550067 (diunduh tanggal 20 Januari 2007)

[12] Puthenpurakal A, Crussell J. Stroke 1: Definition, burden, risk factors and diagnosis. Nursing Times. 2017;**113**(11):43-47

[13] Reitsma MB et al. Spatial, temporal, and demographic patterns in prevalence of smoking tobacco use and attributable disease burden in 204 countries and territories, 1990-2019: A systematic analysis from the Global Burden of Disease Study 2019. Lancet. 2021;**397**: 2337-2360. DOI: 10.1016/ S0140-6736 (21)01169-7

[14] Badan Penelitian dan Pengembangan Kesehatan, "Laporan Nasional Riskesdas 2007," *Lap. Nas. 2007*2007. pp. 1-384 Available from: http://kesga.kemkes.go.id/images/pedoman/Riskesdas 2007 Nasional.pdf

[15] Martini S, Sulistyowati S, Hargono A. Model informasi Kesehatan sebagai Deteksi Dini Kasus Stroke. Surabaya: Lembaga Penelitian Universitas Airlangga; 2008

[16] Kemenkes RI. Laporan Riset Kesehatan Dasar Indonesia 2013. Riskesdas. 2013;**1**:90-93

[17] Kemenkes RI. Laporan Riset Kesehatan Dasar Indonesia 2018. Riskesdas. 2018;**2018**:182-183

[18] Pinto A, Tuttolomondo A, Di Raimondo D, Di Sciacca R, Fernandez P, Di Gati M. A case control study between diabetic and non diabetic subjects with ischemic stroke. International Angiology. 2007;**26**(1):26-32

[19] Kissela BM et al. Epidemiology of ischemic stroke in patients with diabetes: The greater Cincinnati/ Northern Kentucky stroke study. Diabetes Care. 2005;**28**(2):355-359. DOI: 10.2337/diacare.28.2.355

[20] Shah TG, Sutaria JM, Vyas MV. The association between pulmonary hypertension and stroke: A systematic review and meta-analysis. International Journal of Cardiology. 2019;**295**:21-24. DOI: 10.1016/j.ijcard.2019.07.085

[21] Eastwood SV, Tillin T, Chaturvedi N, Hughes AD. Ethnic differences in associations between blood pressure and stroke in South Asian and European men. Hypertension. 2015;**66**(3):481-488. DOI: 10.1161/HYPERTENSIONAHA.115.05672

[22] Roth GA et al. Global burden of cardiovascular diseases and risk factors, 1990 – 2019. Update from the GBD 2019 study. Journal of The American College of Cardiology. 2020;**76**(25):2982-3021. DOI: 10.1016/j.jacc.2020.11.010

[23] Liao CC et al. Impact of diabetes on stroke risk and outcomes: Two nationwide retrospective cohort studies. Medicine. 2015;**94**(52):1-8. DOI: 10.1097/MD.0000000000002282

[24] Boehme AK, Esenwa C, Elkind MSV. Stroke risk factors, genetics, and prevention. Circulation Research. 2017;**120**(3):472-495. DOI: 10.1161/CIRCRESAHA.116.308398

[25] Banerjee C, Moon YP, Paik MC, Rundek T, Mora-McLaughlin C, Vieira JR, et al. Duration of diabetes and risk of ischemic stroke: The Northern Manhattan Study. Stroke. 2012;**43**(5):1 212-1217. DOI: 10.1161/STROKEAHA. 111.641381

[26] Khoury JC et al. Diabetes mellitus: A risk factor for ischemic stroke in a large biracial population. Stroke. 2013;**44**(6): 1500-1504. DOI: 10.1161/STROKEAHA. 113.001318

[27] Kaarisalo MM, Räihä I, Arve S, Lehtonen A. Impaired glucose tolerance as a risk factor for stroke in a cohort of non-institutionalised people aged 70 years. Age and Ageing. 2006;**35**(6): 592-596. DOI: 10.1093/ageing/afl094

[28] Sarwar N et al. Diabetes mellitus, fasting blood glucose concentration, and risk of vascular disease: A collaborative meta-analysis of 102 prospective studies. Lancet. 2010; **375**(9733):2215-2222. DOI: 10.1016/ S0140-6736(10)60484-9

[29] Lau LH, Lew J, Borschmann K, Thijs V, Ekinci EI. Prevalence of diabetes and its effects on stroke outcomes: A meta-analysis and literature review. Journal of Diabetes Investigation. 2019;**10**(3):780-792. DOI: 10.1111/ jdi.12932

[30] Abbafati C et al. Five insights from the Global Burden of Disease Study 2019. Lancet. 2020;**396**:1135-1159

[31] Roy-O'Reilly M, McCullough LD. Age and sex are critical factors in ischemic stroke pathology. Endocrinology. 2018;**159**(8):3120-3131. DOI: 10.1210/ en.2018-00465

[32] Benjamin EJ et al. Heart disease and stroke statistics'2017 update: A report from the American Heart Association. Circulation. 2017;**135**(10):146-603

[33] Teh WL et al. Prevalence of stroke, risk factors, disability and care needs in older adults in Singapore: Results from

the WiSE study. BMJ Open. 2018;**8**(3):1-9. DOI: 10.1136/bmjopen-2017-020285

[34] Rask-Madsen C, King GL. Vascular complications of diabetes: mechanisms of injury and protective factors. Cell Metabolism. 2013;**17**(1):20-33. DOI: 10.1016/j.cmet.2012.11.012

[35] Tun NN, Arunagirinathan G, Pappachan JM. Diabetes mellitus and stroke : A clinical update Diabetes and stroke: Epidemiology. World Journal Diabetes. 2017;**8**(6):235-224. DOI: 10.4239/wjd.v8.i6.235.CITATIONS

[36] Ohiagu FO, Chikezie PC, Chikezie CM. Pathophysiology of diabetes mellitus complications: Metabolic events and control. Biomedical Research and Therapy. 2021;**8**(3):4243-4257. DOI: 10.15419/bmrat.v8i3.663

[37] Ismail L, Materwala H, Al Kaabi J. Association of risk factors with type 2 diabetes: A systematic review. Computational and Structural Biotechnology Journal. 2021;**19**:1759-1785. DOI: 10.1016/j.csbj.2021.03.003

[38] Suastika K, Dwipayana P, Siswadi M, Tuty RA. Age is an Important Risk Factor for Type 2 Diabetes Mellitus and Cardiovascular Diseases. Glucose Tolerance. Croatia: InTech; 2012. DOI: 10.5772/52397

[39] Rachmah Q, Kriengsinyos W, Rojroongwasinkul N, Pongcharoen T. Development and validity of semi-quantitative food frequency questionnaire as a new research tool for sugar intake assessment among Indonesian adolescents. Heliyon. 2021;7(6):e07288. DOI: 10.1016/j.heliyon.2021.e07288

[40] Kementerian Kesehatan RI. Laporan Nasional Riset Kesehatan Dasar 2018. Riskesdas. 2018;**1**:614

[41] Rachmi CN, Jusril H, Ariawan I, Beal T, Sutrisna A. Eating behaviour of

Indonesian adolescents: A systematic review of the literature. Public Health Nutrition. 2020;**24**(Lmic):s84-s97. DOI: 10.1017/S1368980020002876

[42] Usfar AA, Fahmida U. Do Indonesians follow its dietary guidelines? - Evidence related to food consumption, healthy lifestyle, and nutritional status within the period 2000-2010. Asia Pacific Journal of Clinical Nutrition. 2011;**20**(3):484-494. DOI: 10.6133/apjcn.2011.20.3.20

[43] Lowe C et al. The double burden of malnutrition and dietary patterns in rural Central Java, Indonesia. The Lancet Regional Health-Western Pacific. 2021;**14**:100205. DOI: 10.1016/j.lanwpc.2021.100205

[44] Andarwulan N et al. Food consumption pattern and the intake of sugar, salt, and fat in the South Jakarta City—Indonesia. Nutrients. 2021;**13**(4):1-19. DOI: 10.3390/nu13041289

[45] Widijanti A, Ratulangi BT. Pemeriksaan Laboratorium Penderita Diabetes Mellitus. Indonesia: Medika, no. 3, tahun XXIX.; 2003. pp. 167-169

[46] Martini S. Risk Index of Infarct Stroke based on Modifiable Risk Factors [thesis]. Surabaya, Indonesia: Postgraduate Program, Universitas Airlangga; 2010

[47] Berger K, Schulte H, Stögbauer F, Assmann G. Incidence and risk factors for stroke in an occupational cohort: The PROCAM study. Stroke. 1998;**29**(8):1562-1566. DOI: 10.1161/01.STR.29.8.1562

[48] Boden-Albala B et al. Diabetes, fasting glucose levels, and risk of ischemic stroke and vascular events: Findings from the Northern Manhattan Study (NOMAS). Diabetes Care. 2008;**31**(6):1132-1137. DOI: 10.2337/dc07-0797.Additional

[49] O'Donnell MJ et al. Risk factors for ischaemic and intracerebral

haemorrhagic stroke in 22 countries (the INTERSTROKE study): A case-control study. Lancet. 2010;**376**(9735):112-123. DOI: 10.1016/S0140-6736(10)60834-3

[50] Ottenbacher KJ, Ostir GV, Peek MK, Markides KS. Diabetes mellitus as a risk factor for stroke incidence and mortality in Mexican American older adults. The Journals of Gerontology Series A: Biological Sciences and Medical Sciences. 2004;**59**(6):640-645. DOI: 10.1093/gerona/59.6.m640

[51] Munoz-Rivas N et al. Time trends in ischemic stroke among type 2 diabetic and non-diabetic patients: Analysis of the Spanish national hospital discharge data (2003-2012). PLoS One. 2015; **10**(12):1-17. DOI: 10.1371/journal. pone.0145535

[52] Chen R, Ovbiagele B, Feng W. Diabetes and stroke: Epidemiology, pathophysiology, pharmaceuticals and outcomes. The American Journal of the Medical Sciences. 2016;**351**(4):380-386. DOI: 10.1016/j.amjms.2016.01.011

[53] Menon V et al. Impact of baseline glycemic control on residual cardiovascular risk in patients with diabetes mellitus and high-risk vascular disease treated with statin therapy. Journal of the American Heart Association. 2020;**9**(1):1-7. DOI: 10.1161/JAHA.119.014328

[54] Fahimfar N, Khalili D, Mohebi R, Azizi F, Hadaegh F. Risk factors for ischemic stroke; results from 9 years of follow-up in a population based cohort of Iran. BMC Neurology. 2012;**12**:1-7. DOI: 10.1186/1471-2377-12-117

[55] Nomani AZ, Nabi S, Ahmed S, Iqbal M, Rajput HM, Rao S. High HbA1c is associated with higher risk of ischaemic stroke in Pakistani population without diabetes. Stroke and Vascular Neurology. 2016;**1**(3):133-139. DOI: 10.1136/svn-2016-000018

[56] Barasi, M. E. (2009). at a Glance Ilmu Gizi. Jakarta: Erlangga. Page 2. 82

Chapter 9

Aging Associated Specificity in Training Visual Short-Term Memory

Olga Razumnikova and Vladislav Kagan

Abstract

There are numerous data in existence, the computerized cognitive training programs (CCTP) maintain or improve the plasticity of the neural networks in the brain. It is known as well that CCTP reduces the probability of cognitive dysfunctions associated with aging. In the chapter, the age-associated specificity in the temporal dynamics of changes in the visuospatial short-term memory (VSWM, also called visuospatial working memory) is presented. VSWM has been analyzed as there are evidence for age-related decline in visuospatial memory associated with hippocampus atrophy in aging. Memory retrieval decline in older women in comparison with young women while computerized training at home is shown. The elderly achieving results which are comparable to the youngs are determined by significantly increased duration while performing the memory tasks. To reveal factors of the CCTP's efficiency, age-related differences in the attention systems using the Attention Network Test were resolved. In the group of older women, VSWM efficiency is negatively related to the errors of incongruent information selection whereas in young women—to the reaction time while testing. Thus, the success of long-term systematic training of visuospatial memory in old age is strongly related to the high level of executive control.

Keywords: age, visuospatial short-term working memory, memory training, executive control

1. Introduction

The growing part of seniors in population into economically developed countries is associated with a risk of cognitive dysfunctions and brain ischemia due to cardiovascular disease (CVD) that has prompted numerous studies on the mechanisms of brain aging. Age-induced structural and functional changes in the brain including neuronal death, loss of synapses, and dysfunction of neuronal networks relate to such cognitive changes as a decline in the speed of mental activity, inhibitory processes, and short-term memory, including visuospatial short-term memory [1–6].

Aging is a complicated process that has a broad impact on human being in all countries. Aging has some unwelcome consequences to result such as the appearance of neurodegenerative processes and age-related atherosclerotic vascular disruptions which are cause cognitive deficits in elder age [7, 8].

However, there are several important modulating factors that do a preservation impact on cognitive functions in late ontogenesis, which are—education, occupational cognitive activity, locomotor activity, and eating habits. These factors and other conditions in the developmental context are build up compensatory brain resources that form through the lifespan of a person [9, 10]. Aging is a complicated process of the human being. It has some unwelcome consequences to result, such as the appearance of neurodegenerative processes and age-related atherosclerotic vascular disruptions which cause a cognitive deficit in elder age.

A meta-analysis of studies that goals investigation of the forces and trends of cognitive functions, related to various periods of the ontogenesis, shows—there is significant variability of these processes. Consequently, the conclusion of the meta-analysis point to the necessity of further studies aimed to clarify which factors stimulate or prevent cognitive deficits, and what is their weight [10]. The noted variability is due to the fact that almost every age effect is a multicomponent phenomenon, sensitive to the peculiarities of the tasks, the research context, and motivation when doing CCTPs.

Moreover, almost every cognitive task can be performed on the basis of different individual strategies. This means that they are differently associated with aging and include different neural mechanisms for its implementation. Thus, because of the multifactoriality of the research subject, it is difficult to generalize and compare the effects in the studied age groups.

The hypotheses about the role of the plasticity of functional neural networks and lifelong learning in the formation and maintenance of cognitive reserves are widely known. Armed with those ideas, researchers develop CCTP or/and brain training games (BTG). And there are numerous studies of their effect on the preservation of mental health and the prevention of dementia and other cognitive impairments [11–16]. Despite the positive effect described by different authors according to the indicators of motor response and functions of attention and memory [11, 15, 17, 18], accompanied by structural changes with an increase in the mass of gray and white matter of the brain and the reorganization of its functional activity [19, 20], the question remains about the long-term beneficial effect of CCTP. In addition, further researches are warranted to determine the expansion of cognitive-training-related effects to the general state of cognitive activity necessary for daily adaptation [20, 21]. Some researchers to increase the probability of this expansion propose to pay attention to the personalization of a CCTP, and to increase efficiency—to perform the training not individually, but in groups [11]. However, according to another point of view, exactly individualized computerized cognitive training may enhance cognitive self-efficacy in healthy seniors [22].

There are also results showing a positive effect of BTG on cognitive function only in a group of healthy subjects [23]. It should also be noted that some authors point out that different computerized brain training programs work in different ways. The plasticity-based cognitive training programs have a positive effect on cognitive ability, while the computer game training program, which also involves cognitive functions, does not [24].

A meta-analysis reported promising effects of both working memory training and executive functioning training on cognitive functioning in healthy adults aged 60 years and older [25]; albeit, the findings have been contested [26]. A recent analysis of publications on CCTP failed to provide evidence of a significant improvement in cognitive function after computerized cognitive training interventions lasting at least 12 weeks on cognitive function in cognitively healthy people [27]. The authors note that further research is required, possibly longer training, to achieve a sustainable CCTP outcome.

Indeed, 10-year cognitive training data for older people living in the commune show improvements in their cognitive functions not only as a result of subjective assessment, but also in psychometric measurements of reasoning ability or reaction rate, but not memory [18]. It should be noted that there is a lack of scientific evidence for the effectiveness of cognitive training, and perceptions of its benefits are driven by the commercialization of this industry (see e.g., Harrell et al. [28]). Such conflicting points of view require clarification of the reasons for this discrepancy.

There are evidence for age-related atrophy in several brain regions, more often including the hippocampus and prefrontal cortex [29, 30]. The findings suggest that age-related decline in memory can be linked to encoding processes as well as to general cognitive-control operations.

One of the well-known theories to explain the cognitive deficit associated with aging is the theory of "frontal aging" [31, 32], according to which its main cause is the weakening of inhibitory functions during the selection of incongruent information and executive control of problem-solving choice and behavior in general. It was shown that older adults are able to improve inhibition performance through practice [33], and repetition learning is effective in enhancing VSWM in aging and acts through modifications at different stages of stimulus processing [34]. There is evidence for greater interference on a visuospatial compared with a verbal span task (see also Park et al. [35]). The task requires the participant to remember the presented particular blocks. It is believed to involve a number of components important to VSWM—encoding of visual stimuli, maintenance of that information, and memory retrieval. Some studies have already shown that encoding strategies are modified by aging, notably self-initiated strategies [36].

Considering the above-mentioned diversity in opinions regarding the effectiveness of cognitive training, the purpose of our study was to elucidate the age-related characteristics of the temporal dynamics of VSWM and to determine the value of executive control of behavior when testing VSWM.

2. Materials and methods

2.1 Design

Prospective, single-center, single-arm, nonrandomized study conducted at students/listeners of the Novosibirsk State Technical University (NSTU).

2.2 Participants

For investigation of differences in the time dynamics of the effectiveness of VSWM training in dependency of age, we recruited two groups of volunteers. The first group—the elderly—contained 65 women of retirement age (66.3 ± 8.5 years) who studied instruction of the Public Faculty of NSTU. This group had designated as GrE1. The second group—the youngs—contained 94 female students of NSTU's psychology chair (20.1 ± 1.7 years). This group had designated as GrY1.

At the second stage was performed the analysis of the relationship between VSWM and executive control of behavior in the ANT model. These 56 women formed a group designated as GrE2.

The reason for the female composition of the studied groups consisted in the overwhelming majority of the students-retirees (98%) of the Public Faculty are women. Therefore, for comparison VSWM, the group of young participants in the study was also formed only of girls. Moreover, as cerebrovascular accidents were more frequent in women [37], assessing the possibilities of activating their cognitive reserves through VSWM training seems to be practically useful.

2.3 Procedures

For the VSWM, the workout was used a computerized version of the modified "Visual Patterns test" [38]. The program shows a series of randomly generated spatial patterns of blue squares (**Figure 1A**). The presentation of spatial patterns produces in a 6 × 6 matrix. The minimum number of stimuli was 3, the maximum was 13. The pattern of stimuli was displayed for 2 seconds and then disappeared.

According to the instruction, after disappearing the blue-colored spatial pattern, a subject tries to reproduce this pattern by clicking on the unfilled matrix.

The correctly clicked cells turn green (**Figure 1B**), while the wrong clicked cells become red. In case when the reproducing of a pattern is out of time, the whole trial regards as incorrect (**Figure 1C**). In this case, a trial repeats with the pattern of the same number of the blue squares (re-located randomly). The total allowed number of incorrect trials in the one session is limited to 5.

If a trial of reproducing a pattern was successful (i.e., all cells turned green from the first try without any mishits) it regards as correct. In this case, a subject is moved to the next pattern with the increased number of blue squares by 1.

The experimental session overs in two conditions:

1. The number of blue squares in pattern reaches the pre-set maximum [13];

2. A subject reaches the limit of the allowed incorrect trials [5].

One whole session contains 11 trials with 88 blue squares in total.

Each participant was requested to complete 5 sessions of visuospatial memory testing.

The experimental procedure was supported by web-based software that we specially developed. It is available for authorized access at http://psytest.nstu.ru/tests/23/.

An example stimuli presentation to testing the visuospatial working memory (a screenshot from the software that was used in the training):

The efficiency of memory was determined in the percentage of the maximum possible stimuli retrieval—100% reflected the correct reproduction of 88 stimuli presented in 11 trials (using one session).

Instructions for training memory at home were given to students in practical classes in psychology. Students of the Public Faculty—received the instructions in a lecture on the psychophysiology of brain aging, followed by the practice of testing memory in a computer class. Participants were asked to further systematically

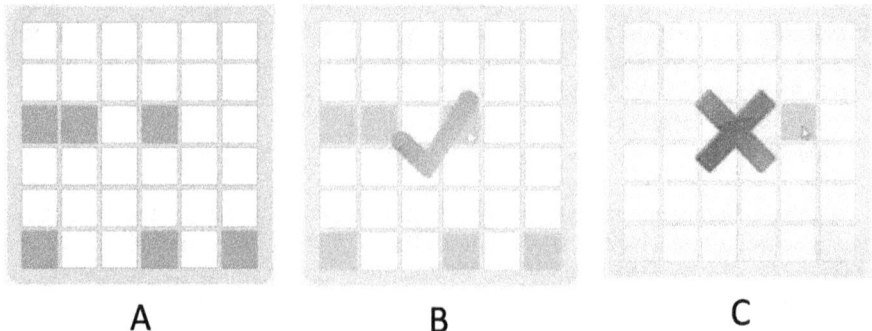

A   **B**   **C**

Figure 1.
Randomly generated spatial pattern—A; correctly clicked cells and correct trial—B; incorrect trial—C.

A   B

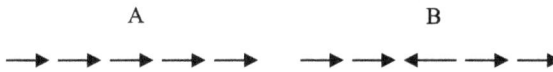

Figure 2.
Stimuli for determining the functions of the executive attention system: A—Congruent, B—Incongruent.

perform the task in order to achieve 80–100% efficiency of VSWM reproduction. The results of all sessions were saved to a database on the university server.

To estimate the function of the executive system of attention was used a computerized method, developed as part of the approach to assessing attention systems (Attention Network Test, ANT) [39] (programmer A.M.Suslov, A.S. 2012617379 dated 16.08.2012). The index of the functiotn of the executive attention system (RTex) was calculated as the difference in response time to the central arrow in the situation of selection of congruent (RTc) (**Figure 2A**) and incongruent (RTnc) (**Figure 2B**) stimuli. The number of errors in response to congruent and incongruent stimuli (Nc and Nnc, respectively) was also recorded.

The software package StatSoft Statistica 13.3.1 Ru AXA805I391121ARCN5-S was used for statistical data processing.

3. Results

3.1 Age differences in visuospatial short-term memory and time dynamic during training

A one-way ANOVA (AGE factor) was used to analyze the effectiveness of memory recall in the first testing session. A significant effect of the AGE factor was found: F (1, 157) = 53.13, p = 0.00000, η2 = 0.25, due to lower values of reproduction in GrE1 compared to GrY1 (50.1 ± 2.0 and 68.7 ± 1.6, respectively). **Table 1** shows the distribution of VSWM efficiency in the first test depending on age, from which it follows that in GrE1 only 16.9% demonstrated retrieval better than 60%, while in GrY1 61.6%. The training criterion in GrY1 already at the first testing reached 28.7%, while in GrE1—only 1.5% (1 person).

The observed decrease in VSWM efficiency in GrE1 compared to GrY1 is consistent with data from other studies of age-related differences in visual-spatial memory [4, 40–43].

The trajectory of the intensity of memory training in two age groups is shown in **Figure 3**—after the first five sessions, the number of participants in training from GrE1 systematically increases compared to GrY1. Analysis of the dynamics of memory retrieval in the first five sessions showed significant effects of the AGE and SESSION factors (F (1, 88) = 34.41; p < 0.00001, η2 = 0.31 and F (3, 264) = 11.44; p < 0.00000, η2 = 0.13, respectively), due to lower memory indices in GrE1 compared to GrY1 (54.0 ± 2.2 and 71.1 ± 1.9) and a similar dynamics in the groups of increase in indices in the 4th and 5th sessions compared to the 1st

Group	Retrieval (%)							
	20–30	30–40	40–50	50–60	60–70	70–80	80–90	90–100
GrE1	3,1	15,4	40,0	24,6	12,3	3,1	0,0	1,5
GrY1	1,1	4,3	7,4	25,5	22,3	10,6	11,7	17,0

Table 1.
The effectiveness of VSWM retrieval in the groups of elderly (GrE1) and young (GrY1) women.

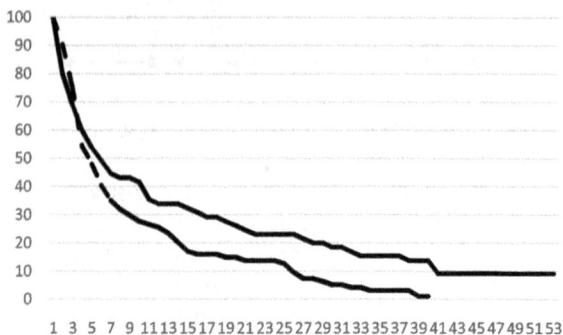

Figure 3.
Change in the number (%) of young (dotted line) and elderly (solid line) participants in memory training depending on the session number (x-axis).

(0.00000 < p < 0.000002 with post hoc analysis of the SESSION effect with Bonferroni correction).

Up to 30 training sessions in GrE1 were performed by 18.5% of the study participants, and in GrY1—only 5.3%. However, this small part of GrY1 achieved an improvement in VSWM retrieval, while GrE1 failed to achieve the criterion required according to the instructions (**Figure 4**).

The observed decrease in the number of participants in cognitive training in GrE1 is similar to that obtained in the course of the Finnish geriatric study aimed at preventing cognitive impairment [44]. Despite the positive effect of long-term training, only a small part of GrE1 achieved it. Therefore, we should agree with the conclusion that home workouts without external control of their implementation are not effective enough [45] for those people who do not have high self-control over their activities.

Five people from GrE1 continued their memory training for over 3 months. The effect of improving their memory in session 87 according to the Wilcoxon criterion was significantly higher than in the first one (p = 0.04) (**Figure 5**), and the average value of reproduction reached the proposed criterion of 80%.

Thus, the internal motivation for starting memory training is insufficient to achieve its effectiveness in GrE1, since most of its participants stop performing the task after only five trials, without achieving the required effect of improving memory. Persistence in VSWM training manifested by a small part of GrE1

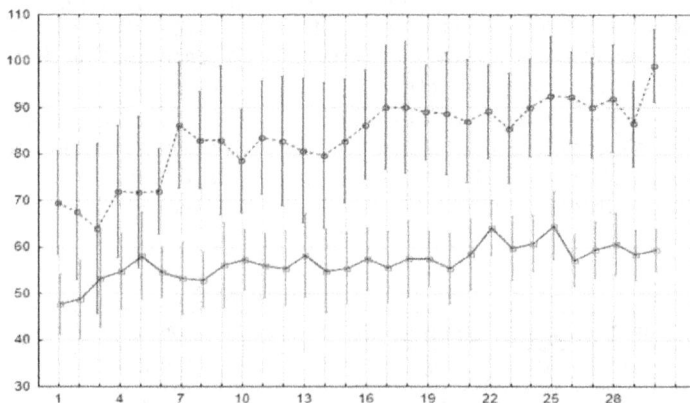

Figure 4.
The efficiency of memory reproduction in groups of young (dotted line) and elderly (solid line) participants in memory training, depending on the session number (x-axis).

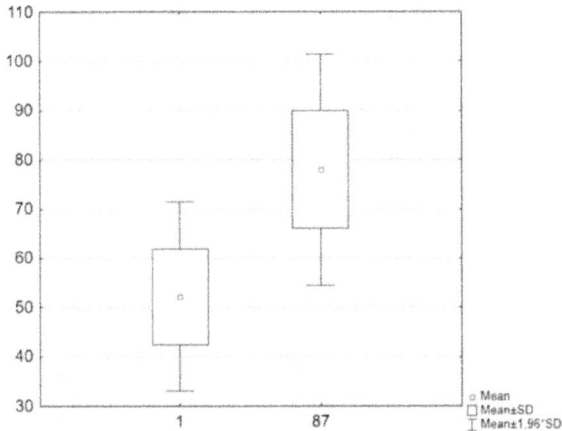

Figure 5.
Memory recall efficiency in the long-term training group during the first test and in the 87th session.

indicates the possibility of achieving a positive effect only when more than 80 sessions are implemented within 3 months, while in GrY1 seven sessions are enough to increase the effectiveness of VSWM.

The effectiveness of performing VSWM tasks is associated with the influence of practice and interference processes, each of which has an age specificity, and the combination of a higher learning rate with more pronounced interference in young people than in old age can determine the individual effectiveness of cognitive training [43, 46].

Several factors are also known to support long-term cognitive training. These include the possession of high behavior control, intrinsic motivation to achieve a goal, and interest in the performed activity, including due to the awareness of the development of cognitive deficits [22, 28, 47]. Previously, it was shown that when assessing motivational inducers of behavior, older women single out cognitive training as a priority in maintaining their health; however, only 8% of this group actually consistently participated in cognitive training using a battery of computerized techniques [48]. Consequently, the different age dynamics of memory training noted by us can be associated with the dominance of the learning potential in GrY1 and motivation to perform the task in GrE1.

It is believed that aging is associated with the effect of increased costs of cognitive interaction and increased effort required to achieve a high level of task performance [49, 50]. Therefore, older people become more selective and economical in the use of cognitive resources, which is reflected in a decrease in intrinsic motivation to participate in predictably complex cognitive activities. Apparently, therefore, the lack of visible success after the first training sessions causes them to refuse further activities. Individualized cognitive training with feedback that reinforces subjective assessments of change can help to improve cognitive self-esteem in older adults [22], and success can help to reduce perceptions of difficulties and become more willing to participate in cognitive activities [50].

It has been shown that the effectiveness of cognitive training can be increased due to involvement in activities and increased motivation through learning cognitive control using play procedures or nonplay learning [51]. Improving visual memory is possible through the application of a strategy for controlling attention and directing it to target memory components [40].

In this regard, the next stage of our study was devoted to elucidating the relationship between VSWM and executive attention control.

3.2 Role of executive control in the efficiency of the visuospatial short-term memory

This stage of the research was devoted to the analysis of the relationship between VSWM and executive control of behavior in the ANT model.

VSWM assessment was carried out according to the method described in clause 3.1 above.

The indicators of attention and memory in the studied groups are shown in **Table 2**. According to the intergroup comparison, all indicators differed significantly—GrE2 was characterized by lower memory values, but a large number of errors and a longer reaction time when testing executive control of attention.

By the correlation analysis of the ratio of VSWM and attention indices in each group a negative relationship was found between the VSWM efficiency with Nnc in GrE2 ($r = -0.31$, $p < 0.02$) and with RTnc ($r = -0.35$, $p < 0.01$) in GrY2.

Consequently, in GrE2, the memorization efficiency is associated with the control of the accuracy of information selection, and in GrY2, with the information selection rate.

The relationship between executive control and working memory, including VSWM, is well known [52–54], but continues to attract the interest of researchers since their age-related changes determine preservation of intellectual abilities and quality of life during aging [55]. According to the results of tomographic studies, cortical thinning of the right anterior cingulate and middle frontal gyri showed progression from mild cognitive impairment (MCI) to Alzheimer's disease (AD) [52]. Since these brain structures are associated with such WM functions as the selection of information relevant for memorization and inhibition of irrelevant information, tracking executive function performance can be a useful tool to assess an individual's cognitive abilities in older adults as well as a strong predictor of progression from MCI to AD. In this regard, executive attention control training is included in complex multimodal cognitive training programs for patients with MCI [56]. Our data are consistent with these views, indicating a positive relationship between the effectiveness of the executive functions of attention and VSWM. It is noteworthy that if in GrY2 a high speed of information selection is required for successful reproduction of VSWM, then in GrE2 the predominant role is played by the selection accuracy with inhibition of irrelevant stimuli. Consequently, regardless of the general slowdown in the rate of cognitive processes characteristic of old age [5, 6, 37, 57], such a reorganization of information selection is possible, in particular, through the strategy of redistribution of directed attention [40] or modifications at different stages of stimulus processing [34], which provides an effective VSWM.

Thus, according to the results of the second part of the study, the preservation of executive control of attention should be recognized as a necessary condition for successful long-term VSWM training in GrE1.

Group	VSWM	ANT				
		Nc	Nnc	RTc	RTnc	RTex
GrE2	67.9 ± 7.4***	0.3 ± 0.5*	3.5 ± 4.3***	841 ± 159***	952 ± 157***	111 ± 56**
GrY2	82.5 ± 7.6	0.1 ± 0.3	1.5 ± 2.3	541 ± 77	634 ± 90	93 ± 42

*<0.05.
**<0.01.
***<0.001.

Table 2.
Indicators of attention and memory in the elderly group (GrE2) and young group (GrY2).

4. Conclusion

The results obtained in our study show that despite the initially lower VSWM indicators in older women than in younger women, long-term (more than 3 months) training allows you to achieve a result comparable to that of young women; and because of that to achieve effectiveness in cognitive training in the elderly internal control of behavior is crucial.

Indeed, according to the results of the experiment to determine the ratio of VSWM and psychometric assessment of the functions of executive attention, the relationship between VSWM and exactitude processing of information selection in the elderly group is established.

Therefore, achieving an improvement in VSWM in old age requires persistence and a prolonged training period, which is provided by executive control of cognitive activity. The success of cognitive training at home for the individual execution of computerized programs is possible in the presence of internal motivation and high executive control of behavior.

Hence, memory decline as a consequence of cerebrovascular disease can be compensated by cognitive training and psychological support of insufficiently effective initially obtained results. Such support is natively possible in group of cognitive training programs at neurorehabilitation centers. Also, such a psychological support can be realized in computerized training programs in the form of feedback to emotional reinforcement. Especially when the current result are not satisfied and motivation for continue training are insufficient.

Acknowledgements

This study was supported by the Ministry of Science and Higher Education of Russian Federation (project No. FSUN-2020-0009). Conflict of Interest: The authors declare that they have no conflicts of interest.

Author details

Olga Razumnikova* and Vladislav Kagan
Novosibirsk State Technical University, Novosibirsk, Russia

*Address all correspondence to: razoum@mail.ru

IntechOpen

References

[1] Harada CN, Natelson Love MC, Triebel KL. Normal Cognitive Aging. Clinics in Geriatric Medicine. 2013; **29**(4):737-752

[2] Hertzog C, Kramer AF, Wilson RS, Lindenberger U. Enrichment effects on adult cognitive development: Can the functional capacity of older adults be preserved and enhanced? Psychological Science in the Public Interest. 2008;**9**(1):1-65

[3] Hubert V, Beaunieux H, Chételat G, Platel H, Landeau B, Viader F, et al. Age-related changes in the cerebral substrates of cognitive procedural learning. Human Brain Mapping. 2009;**30**(4):1374-1386

[4] Perrochon A, Mandigout S, Petruzzellis S, Soria Garcia N, Zaoui M, Berthoz A, et al. The influence of age in women in visuo-spatial memory in reaching and navigation tasks with and without landmarks. Neuroscience Letters. 2018;**684**:13-17

[5] Razumnikova OM. Effects of aging brain and activation methods of its compensatory resources. Advances in Physiological Sciences. 2015;**46**(2):3-16 (In Russian)

[6] Salthouse T. Consequences of age-related cognitive declines. Annual Review of Psychology. 2012;**63**(1):201-226

[7] Tarasova IV, Trubnikova OA, Razumnikova OM. Plasticity of brain functional systems as a compensator resource in normal and pathological aging associated with atherosclerosis. Ateroscleroz. 2020;**16**(1):59-67 (In Russian)

[8] Martinic-Popovic I, Simundic A-M, Dukic L, Lovrencic-Huzjan A, Popovic A, Seric V, et al. The association of inflammatory markers with cerebral vasoreactivity and carotid atherosclerosis in transient ischaemic attack. Clinical Biochemistry. 2014;**47**(16-17):182-186

[9] Chen P, Goedert KM, Murray E, Kelly K, Ahmeti S, Barrett AM. Spatial bias and right hemisphere function: Sex-specific changes with aging. Journal of the International Neuropsychological Society. 2011;**17**(3):455-462

[10] Rut C, Jose B, Antonieta N. Age-related cognitive changes: The importance of modulating factors. Journal of Geriatric Medicine Gerontology. 2018;**4**(2):48

[11] Kelly ME, Loughrey D, Lawlor BA, Robertson IH, Walsh C, Brennan S. The impact of cognitive training and mental stimulation on cognitive and everyday functioning of healthy older adults: A systematic review and meta-analysis. Ageing Research Reviews. 2014;**15**:28-43

[12] Mahncke HW, Bronstone A, Merzenich MM. Brain plasticity and functional losses in the aged: Scientific bases for a novel intervention. Progress in Brain Research. 2006;**157**:81-109

[13] Campos-Magdaleno M, Leiva D, Pereiro AX, Lojo-Seoane C, Mallo SC, Facal D, et al. Changes in visual memory in mild cognitive impairment: A longitudinal study with CANTAB. Psychological Medicine. 2020;**7**:1-11

[14] McCallum S, Boletsis C. A taxonomy of serious games for dementia. In: Schouten B, Fedtke S, Bekker T, Schijven M, Gekker A, editors. Games for Health. Wiesbaden: Springer Fachmedien Wiesbaden; 2013. pp. 219-232

[15] Edwards JD, Phillips CB, O'Connor ML, O'Brien JL, Hudak EM, Nicholson JS. Applying the health belief model to quantify and investigate expectations for computerized cognitive

training. Journal of Cognitive Enhancement. 2021;**5**(1):51-61

[16] Edwards JD, Fausto BA, Tetlow AM, Corona RT, Valdés EG. Systematic review and meta-analyses of useful field of view cognitive training. Neuroscience & Biobehavioral Reviews. 2018;**84**:72-91

[17] Giuli C, Papa R, Lattanzio F, Postacchini D. The effects of cognitive training for elderly: Results from my mind project. Rejuvenation Research. 2016;**19**(6):485-494

[18] Rebok GW, Ball K, Guey LT, Jones RN, Kim H-Y, King JW, et al. Ten-year effects of the advanced cognitive training for independent and vital elderly cognitive training trial on cognition and everyday functioning in older adults. Journal of the American Geriatrics Society. 2014;**62**(1):16-24

[19] Jockwitz C, Caspers S, Lux S, Eickhoff SB, Jütten K, Lenzen S, et al. Influence of age and cognitive performance on resting-state brain networks of older adults in a population-based cohort. Cortex. 2017;**89**:28-44

[20] Nguyen L, Murphy K, Andrews G. Immediate and long-term efficacy of executive functions cognitive training in older adults: A systematic review and meta-analysis. Psychological Bulletin. 2019;**145**(7):698-733

[21] JIV B, JMJ M, Ridderinkhof KR. Brain training in progress: A review of trainability in healthy seniors. Frontiers in Human Neuroscience. 2012;**6**:183

[22] Goghari VM, Krzyzanowski D, Yoon S, Dai Y, Toews D. Attitudes and beliefs toward computerized cognitive training in the general population. Frontiers in Psychology. 2020;**11**:503

[23] Al-Thaqib A, Al-Sultan F, Al-Zahrani A, Al-Kahtani F, Al-Regaiey K, Iqbal M, et al. Brain training games enhance cognitive function in healthy subjects. Medical Science Monitor Basic Research. 2018;**24**:63-69

[24] Mahncke HW, DeGutis J, Levin H, Newsome MR, Bell MD, Grills C, et al. A randomized clinical trial of plasticity-based cognitive training in mild traumatic brain injury. Brain. 2021;**144**(7):1994-2008

[25] Karbach J, Verhaeghen P. Making working memory work: A meta-analysis of executive-control and working memory training in older adults. Psychological Science. 2014;**25**(11):2027-2037

[26] Melby-Lervåg M, Hulme C. Is working memory training effective? A meta-analytic review. Developmental Psychology. 2013;**49**(2):270-291

[27] Gates NJ, Rutjes AW, Di Nisio M, Karim S, Chong L-Y, March E, et al. Computerised cognitive training for 12 or more weeks for maintaining cognitive function in cognitively healthy people in late life. Cochrane Dementia and Cognitive Improvement Group, editor. Cochrane Database of Systematic Reviews. 2020;**2**(2):CD012277

[28] Harrell ER, Kmetz B, Boot WR. Is cognitive training worth it? exploring individuals' willingness to engage in cognitive training. Journal of Cognition Enhancement. 2019;**3**(4):405-415

[29] Fjell AM, Walhovd KB, Fennema-Notestine C, McEvoy LK, Hagler DJ, Holland D, et al. One-year brain atrophy evident in healthy aging. Journal of Neuroscience. 2009;**29**(48):15223-15231

[30] Nyberg L, Salami A, Andersson M, Eriksson J, Kalpouzos G, Kauppi K, et al. Longitudinal evidence for diminished frontal cortex function in aging. Proceedings of the National Academy of Sciences. 2010;**107**(52):22682-22686

[31] Denburg NL, Hedgcock WM. Age-associated executive dysfunction, the prefrontal cortex, and complex decision making. Aging and Decision Making. 2015:79-101

[32] West RL. An application of prefrontal cortex function theory to cognitive aging. Psychological Bulletin. 1996;**120**(2):272-292

[33] Wilkinson AJ, Yang L. Inhibition plasticity in older adults: Practice and transfer effects using a multiple task approach. Neural Plasticity. 2016; **2016**:1-12

[34] Tagliabue CF, Assecondi S, Cristoforetti G, Mazza V. Learning by task repetition enhances object individuation and memorization in the elderly. Scientific Reports. 2020;**10**(1): 19957

[35] Park DC, Lautenschlager G, Hedden T, Davidson NS, Smith AD, Smith PK. Models of visuospatial and verbal memory across the adult life span. Psychology and Aging. 2002;**17**(2):299-320

[36] Craik FI. Changes in memory with normal aging: A functional view. Advances in Neurology. 1990;**51**:201-205

[37] Calatayud E, Salavera C, Gómez-Soria I. Cognitive Differences in the Older Adults Living in the General Community: Gender and Mental Occupational State Study. Int J Environ Res Public Health. 17 Mar 2021;**18**(6):3106. DOI: 10.3390/ ijerph18063106. PMID: 33802961; PMCID: PMC8002664.99

[38] Della Sala S, Gray C, Baddeley A, Allamano N, Wilson L. Pattern span: A tool for unwelding visuo–spatial memory. Neuropsychologia. 1999;**37**(10):1189-1199

[39] Fan J, McCandliss BD, Sommer T, Raz A, Posner MI. Testing the efficiency and independence of attentional networks. Journal of Cognitive Neuroscience. 2002;**14**(3):340-347

[40] Allen RJ, Atkinson AL, Nicholls LAB. Strategic prioritisation enhances young and older adults' visual feature binding in working memory. Quarterly Journal of Experimental Psychology. 2021;**74**(2):363-376

[41] Beigneux K, Plaie T, Isingrini M. Aging effect on visual and spatial components of working memory. International Journal of Aging & Human Development. 2007;**65**(4):301-314

[42] Rhodes S, Parra MA, Logie RH. Ageing and feature binding in visual working memory: The role of presentation time. Quarterly Journal of Experimental Psychology. 2016;**69**(4): 654-668

[43] Rowe G, Hasher L, Turcotte J. Age differences in visuospatial working memory. Psychology and Aging. 2008;**23**(1):79-84

[44] Turunen M, Hokkanen L, Bäckman L, Stigsdotter-Neely A, Hänninen T, Paajanen T, et al. Computer-based cognitive training for older adults: Determinants of adherence. Ginsberg SD, editor. PLoS One. 2019;**14**(7):e0219541

[45] Lampit A, Hallock H, Valenzuela M. Computerized cognitive training in cognitively healthy older adults: A systematic review and meta-analysis of effect modifiers. Gandy S, editor. PLoS Medicine. 2014;**11**(11):e1001756

[46] Razumnikova O. Age effect on relationships between inhibitory functions of executive attention system and visual memory. Experimental Psychology (Russia). 2019;**12**(2):61-74

[47] Mohammed S, Flores L, Deveau J, Cohen Hoffing R, Phung CM, Parlett C,

et al. The benefits and challenges of implementing motivational features to boost cognitive training outcome. Journal of Cognition of Enhancement. 2017;**1**(4):491-507

[48] Razumnikova OM, Asanova NV. Motivational inductors of behavior as reserves of successful aging. Advances in Gerontology. 2019;**9**(3):361-365

[49] Hess TM. Selective engagement of cognitive resources: Motivational influences on older adults' cognitive functioning. Perspectives on Psychological Science. 2014;**9**(4):388-407

[50] Hess TM, Lothary AF, O'Brien EL, Growney CM, DeLaRosa J. Predictors of engagement in young and older adults: The role of specific activity experience. Psychology and Aging. 2021;**36**(2):131-142

[51] Vervaeke J, Hoorelbeke K, Baeken C, Van Looy J, Koster EHW. Transfer and motivation after cognitive control training for remitted depression in healthy sample. Journal of Cognitive Enhancement. 2020;**4**(1):49-61

[52] Kirova A-M, Bays RB, Lagalwar S. Working memory and executive function decline across normal aging, mild cognitive impairment, and Alzheimer's disease. BioMed Research International. 2015;**2015**:1-9

[53] Miyake A, Friedman NP, Rettinger DA, Shah P, Hegarty M. How are visuospatial working memory, executive functioning, and spatial abilities related? A latent-variable analysis. Journal of Experimental Psychology: General. 2001;**130**(4):621-640

[54] Wang L, Bolin J, Lu Z, Carr M. Visuospatial working memory mediates the relationship between executive functioning and spatial ability. Frontiers in Psychology. 2018;**9**:2302

[55] Borella E, Cantarella A, Joly E, Ghisletta P, Carbone E, Coraluppi D, et al. Performance-based everyday functional competence measures across the adult lifespan: The role of cognitive abilities. International Psychogeriatrics. 2017;**29**(12):2059-2069

[56] Tsolaki M, Kounti F, Agogiatou C, Poptsi E, Bakoglidou E, Zafeiropoulou M, et al. Effectiveness of nonpharmacological approaches in patients with mild cognitive impairment. Neurodegenerative Diseases. 2011;**8**(3):138-145

[57] Eckert. Age-related changes in processing speed: Unique contributions of cerebellar and prefrontal cortex. Frontiers in Human Neuroscience. 2010;**4**:10

Chapter 10

Stroke Rehabilitation and Occupational Therapy in Low Resource Settings

Tecla Mlambo, Yvonne Pfavai, Faith R. Chimusoro and Farayi Kaseke

Abstract

The long-term complications of stroke interfere with function, and the level of disability varies based on the type of stroke, location, and the extent of damage. Rehabilitation services are important in the recovery of stroke patients, but not all survivors have access to the services especially in low resourced settings where accessibility and economic challenges are the major barriers. Inadequate fulfilment of stroke survivors' rehabilitation needs contribute to poor functional outcomes and slow recovery. The objectives of this chapter is therefore to give an overview of stroke and stroke rehabilitation with specific emphasis on occupational therapy, discuss the activities and areas of participation considered important by stroke patients, stroke patients' needs and perceived fulfilment of these needs in order to provide targeted interventions. Data to inform the chapter is based on research done in a low resource setting. The perceived important activities and participation areas, and the needs of stroke patients are discussed in light of literature on the subject and findings from the studies done in Zimbabwe.

Keywords: stroke, rehabilitation, occupational therapy, activities, functional outcomes, participation areas, stroke survivor needs, ICF

1. Introduction

1.1 Overview of stroke

Stroke is an insult to the brain tissue caused by a sudden interruption to the blood supply to the brain [1]. Sacco et al. gave an elaborate definition of stroke as a neurological deficit attributed to an acute focal injury of the central nervous system (CNS) by a vascular cause, including cerebral infarction, intra-cerebral haemorrhage (ICH), and subarachnoid haemorrhage (SAH) [2]. Stroke is highly prevalent and a second major cause of death and disability worldwide [2–4]. Stroke is a leading cause of dementia and depression. It can be classified on the basis of its aetiology as either ischaemic (87%) or haemorrhagic (13%) [5]. Ischaemic stroke results from occlusion of a cerebral artery which can be thrombotic or atherosclerotic (50%), embolic (25%) and micro-artery occlusion (lacunar stroke or infarcts) (25%) [5]. Haemorrhagic stroke is caused mainly by spontaneous rupture of blood vessels or aneurysms or secondary to trauma [5]. Early definitions of stroke and transient ischemic attack (TIA) focused on the duration of symptoms and signs. However, Sacco et al. [2], noted that use of clinical observations and modern brain imaging showed that the duration and reversibility of brain ischemia is variable. Brain tissue that is deprived of needed nutrients can, in some patients, survive without permanent injury for a considerable period of time, that is, several hours or even, rarely, days, while in most other individuals, irreversible damage (infarction) occurs quickly [2].

There has been a rise in the prevalence of stroke related disability in many countries [6]. A rise in the incidence of stroke in Zimbabwe from 31/100,000 to 57/100,000 in a decade was reported with fatality rates ranging from 22 to 58% at one month following stroke reported in Zimbabwe and other African studies [7].

The risk factors for stroke are generally similar to those for coronary heart diseases and other vascular diseases [4]. High blood pressure is one of the leading primary and secondary modifiable risk factors [5]. The other risk factors for stroke include smoking, low physical activity levels, unhealthy diet, abdominal obesity, diabetes and excessive consumption of alcohol [4]. Effective prevention strategies should include targeting the key modifiable risk factors such as hypertension, elevated lipids and diabetes.

Clinical manifestations of each stroke differ based on the part and side of the brain affected, extent of the lesion and the person's general health. Some of the effects of stroke include numbness, weakness or paralysis on one side of the body opposite the side of the brain affected, slurred speech, difficulty thinking of words or understanding other people, confusion, sudden blurred vision or sight loss, being unsteady on your feet and severe headache [8]. Concerning the stroke warning signs, numbness on one side was surprisingly identified as the commonest warning (44%) while unspecified pain was the least cited (11%) in one of the studies [9]. Stroke can also result in psychological problems such as depression, anxiety, feeling helpless and thoughts of death or suicide, trouble sleeping and feelings of worthlessness [10]. In general, a right cerebrovascular accident may result in left hemiplegia or hemiparesis, difficulties with visuo-spatial memory, neglect of the left side of the body, poor judgement, and impulsivity, while a left cerebrovascular accident may cause right hemiplegia or hemiparesis, apraxia, and aphasia due to the location of the Broccas' and Wernicke's areas [11].

Stroke was associated with 43.7 million disability-adjusted life years annually around the world [5]. It is one of the most common neurological diseases in the black African and the leading cause of adult neurological admissions in West African sub-region, constituting up to 65% of such admissions [9]. Globally, 70% of strokes and 87% of both stroke-related deaths and disability-adjusted life years occur in low- and middle-income countries [4]. Approximately 60% of stroke patients acquire permanent disabilities and experience limitations in terms of mobility, vision, voice, speech, swallowing (dysphagia) and sexual function globally [4]. Stroke can cause multiple impairments which might need a variety of rehabilitation interventions [12]. Motor impairment is the most common deficit after stroke and the motor deficits increase fall risks and fall-related injuries. This in turn significantly affects the patients' mobility, participation in their activities of daily living, social events and other occupational performance areas [13].

Stroke is a leading cause of functional impairments; with 20% of survivors requiring institutional care after three months and 15–30% being permanently disabled [14]. Many stroke patients experience activity limitation, restricted social participation, and psychological issues such as anxiety and depression some years after having stroke [15]. Approximately 65% of stroke patients are dependent on others to help them with everyday activities and the quality of life 2–5 years after stroke has been reported by many stroke survivors as poor [15].

Several researchers have studied the stroke survivor's physical, social, psychological and emotional needs [16–19]. Although most stroke patients receive rehabilitation, the lifelong need for care of stroke patients with disabilities has not been fully explored [17]. Despite calls for comprehensive stroke services to address long-term needs of patients, there had been little investigation of the perceived needs of stroke survivors in the long term or what determines such needs [20]. This area lacked a systematic approach to problem identification, had a poor evidence base, and was not underpinned by sound theoretical concepts hence there was need for further research in the area [15]. Similarly, needs of caregivers for stroke patients need further exploration.

1.2 Stroke rehabilitation and occupational therapy

Stroke Rehabilitation is a progressive, dynamic and goal-orientated process aimed at enabling a person with impairment as a result of stroke to reach their optimal physical, cognitive, emotional, communicative, social and functional activity level [21]. Stroke rehabilitation begins in the acute care hospital after the person's overall condition has been stabilised, often within 24–48 hours after the stroke [22]. Stroke rehabilitation plays a vital role in lessening the effects of impairments and activity limitations, and in facilitating the return to active participation in community life and economic self-sufficiency after the stroke [12]. Internationally recognised best practice in the early management and rehabilitation of individuals following stroke includes collaborative and multidisciplinary assessment and treatment by a coordinated team of health care professionals [23]. A collaborative approach improves quality of life in stroke patients [12].

In the first weeks and months of recovery, the goals of rehabilitation are to help survivors become as independent as possible and to attain the best possible quality of life [21]. Although rehabilitation may not reverse the brain damage, it can substantially help people achieve the best possible long-term outcomes [22] through various ways that include facilitation of neuroplasticity of the brain. Rehabilitation is especially crucial during the early stages of recovery to regain independence when patients have little or no control over their affected muscles [22].

As part of stroke rehabilitation, occupational therapy (OT) involves the use of activities or training to improve or maintain the ability to live independently and cope with daily life for people with stroke [16]. The philosophy of occupational therapy is based on the concept that all humans have a need to become engaged in occupations [24], and that need is present even after stroke. Therefore, the role of the occupational therapist is to facilitate the patient's continued participation in meaningful and purposeful daily activities and adaptation to the patient's changed status. These occupations (all goal-directed engagement in self-care, work or leisure activities) can be termed as activities and participation areas in the International Classification of Functioning, Disability and Health (ICF) terminology [25]. According to the ICF framework, stroke results in activity limitation and participation restriction [26]. The ICF is a globally agreed framework and classification to define the spectrum of problems in the functioning of patients [27]. The ICF was also shown to be an essential tool for identifying and measuring efficacy and effectiveness of rehabilitation services [28]. Using the ICF takes a biopsychosocial approach which addresses the quality of life gap which is often left in favour of quantity of life.

Occupational Therapy in general, focuses on the assessment and treatment of individuals who are limited by physical injury or illness, psychosocial dysfunction, developmental or learning disabilities, or the ageing process through the use of purposeful activity and adaptive equipment and technology in order to maximise independence, prevent disability and maintain health [29]. Occupational therapists play a crucial role in the rehabilitation of stroke patients as they are experts at training patients to relearn complex bodily movements and avoid complications that could derail their progress later [30]. Occupational therapy is concerned with promoting health and wellbeing through participation in activities of everyday life and this is done by modifying the occupations and the environment in a therapeutic way to better support participation [23]. Occupational therapists also employ neurophysiologically based handling techniques meant to facilitate neuroplasticity of the brain. In some instances, occupational therapists can teach compensatory strategies when the old ways of functioning are no longer possible [30]. Therefore, occupational therapy for stroke includes interventions for physical, social, psychological and cognitive impairments [30]. The role of occupational therapists in stroke rehabilitation is particularly important because they focus on functional outcomes and getting clients back to doing everyday activities [11] which is usually unique to the profession. It is important that the interventions suit a patient's needs [30].

The period of receiving services in stroke rehabilitation depends on the severity of disability and specific needs of the stroke survivor, although it has been proved that a great deal of stroke recovery occur within the first six months to a year following the onset of the stroke [31]. Occupational therapists work collaboratively with the patient to establish the impact of stroke on their performance of daily tasks, including personal care, domestic tasks, work and leisure activities; and in formulating a goal-focused program to develop the required skills for participation in daily life [23]. Given the variability in stroke complications, occupational therapists need to have a wide repertoire of techniques to help each client [11]. The treatment techniques in occupational therapy may include using occupational tasks to help improve cognitive abilities, teaching adaptations to meaningful activities to keep the client involved, and using task-specific movement to help with range of motion and motor control [11]. The occupational therapist can provide a patient with an assistive device or adjustments and adaptations in the environment, for example, in a patient's home. This enables the patient to perform his/her ADLs independently and also dealing with other emotional or social issues that may result from stroke [30].

The occupational therapy process for stroke patients begins with an assessment of the patient's roles, tasks and activities that are important for the patient [30]. An assessment is conducted to understand the impact of changes in motor function, sensation, coordination, visual perception, and cognition on the stroke patients and on the capacity to manage daily life tasks [23]. Assessment is also used to identify areas of individual and environmental difficulties and to enable patient-centred goal setting with the participation of both the patient and the caregiver [23]. The occupational therapist will then assess the ability to perform the roles, tasks and activities and if a limitation or restriction in some area is found, the occupational therapist will identify the performance components and craft the solution or intervention meant to restore, improve or maintain patient's maximum level of performance [30]. Some of the performance components may include neuromuscular, cognitive and perceptual, language and psychosocial problems.

The occupational therapy interventions should therefore be able to address the patient's needs and be provided in both the acute and rehabilitation phases [30]. For some stroke survivors, rehabilitation will be an on-going process to maintain and refine skills and could involve working with occupational therapists and other specialists in that field for months or even years after the stroke [22].

2. Activities and areas of participation considered important by stroke patients

In order to adequately address challenges stroke patients face, there is need to identify the activities and areas of participation they consider important. This section is therefore based on a study done in Zimbabwe which sought to find out the activities and areas of participation considered important by stroke patients, the level of difficulty experienced in carrying out these activities and the reasons for attaching importance to these areas [32]. The study was cross sectional descriptive in nature and was done with 40 stroke patients consecutively selected as they came for their reviews at an outpatient stroke clinic at a central hospital in Zimbabwe [33]. An interview questionnaire adapted from the ICF checklist version 2.1a clinician form was administered by the researchers with consent after ethical approval (JREC....). Excluded were patients with significant cognitive and language impairments as it would have been difficult to communicate with them. In the study, 25 were female and 15 were male. Participants' ages ranged from 34 to 81 years with the 50–59 years age group being the mode. These demographic characteristics are consistent with a study done by Mlambo et al. [34], which was done in South Africa and the participants' ages ranged from 32 to 81 with a mean age of 52 years. The activities and areas of participation assessed during the study were obtained from the domains in the ICF checklist as alluded to earlier.

2.1 Mobility and hand function

Half of the patients reported severe difficulty in lifting and carrying objects, while 43 and 38% of participants experienced complete and severe difficulties in fine hand use respectively [32]. About 20% had flexion contractures of the elbow and wrist joints of the affected side. These difficulties were due to the condition (stroke) which causes disturbances in muscle tone and loss of selective and isolated movements in the hand and arm [35] and this hinders execution of functional movements [36]. Thirty three percent of the participants had moderate difficulty in walking and used mobility aids while 20% had complete difficulty [32]. Half of the participants reported experiencing complete difficulty in using transportation like cars or buses. On driving, only 18 participants were drivers and 78% of them reported complete difficulty in the area [32].

On importance attached to these domains, all participants considered fine hand use and walking important, while 98% considered being able to use transportation important [32]. However, it was noted that none of the participants who were drivers had driving addressed by their therapist. Driving rehabilitation is an area that has not been fully explored by OTs in Zimbabwe. Driving is an important ADL and many stroke patients who were driving prior to their stroke wished to resume driving as noted by Kneebone and Lincoln [37]. A study by Duncan et al. [38] found that hand function and mobility were some of the key areas considered important by stroke patients.

2.2 Self-care

Half of the participants in the study reported severe difficulties in dressing, 33% had moderate to severe difficulties in grooming while 65% had severe difficulty in bathing themselves [32]. About 73% had no difficulty in feeding and this can be explained by the exclusion of patients with speech and cognitive problems in the study. Speech and cognitive problems are often associated with feeding problems. Thirty three percent did not experience any difficulties in toileting while the remainder had mild to severe difficulties and used sanitary wear or were catheterised [32].

All aspects of self-care were considered as very important by all participants as they viewed these activities crucial for human survival [32]. This was also noted in a study by Aberg et al. [39] where the participants valued their independence in self-care activities.

2.3 Domestic life

In Chimusoro's study [32], 78 and 75% of participants had complete difficulties in acquisition of goods and services, and preparing meals respectively. About half of the participants considered being able to prepare meals important, while 32% consisting mainly of male participants and elderly female participants did not view it as important since they had their meals prepared for them by caregivers. On doing housework, all male participants considered it as not applicable to them. This is common in the Zimbabwean and most African cultures where most if not all men, do not consider household chores as part of their ADLs. Therefore it would be irrelevant to engage a male patient in therapy sessions focusing on retraining household chores unless found necessary during the assessment process. The same notion applied to the elderly female patients who had long stopped doing those chores before suffering a stroke. These duties were done for them by children, grandchildren and/or caregivers [32]. This is where the aspect of interdependence is seen in the African culture. The elderly in Africa usually end up living with their children and grandchildren as compared to the Western culture where the elderly can be living alone and independence in home maintenance tasks becomes an important aspect of their lives.

2.4 Interpersonal interactions and relationships

All the participants did not have any difficulties in basic interpersonal interactions, formal and informal interactions [32]. Participants considered these areas important. However, 10 and 4% had mild and moderate difficulties in intimate relationships respectively. They attributed their problems in sexual function to their condition and felt it hindered maximum enjoyment of intimate relationships. They viewed their intimate relationships as important but were reluctant to share this with their therapist since they were not aware that the issue could be addressed in occupational therapy. Resumption of sexual activity for stroke patients is very important as cited by Edmans, although they may fail to articulate this to the therapist [40].

2.5 Major life areas

In this domain remunerative employment was not applicable to half of the participants as some were retired and some did not work prior to suffering the stroke. For the remaining half they reported complete difficulty and had not yet returned to their previous jobs. This is consistent with the findings by D'Alisa et al. [41] in which 40% had severe restrictions in employment issues. About 95% of patients to whom employment was applicable considered it as very important [41].

About 33% had moderate difficulties in economic self-sufficiency as they had financial problems due to their unemployment status. All the participants considered being self-sufficient important. In D'Alisa et al. [41], 15% had moderate to severe restrictions in economic self-sufficiency. This difference may be due to lack of a national social security system that cushions persons with disabilities in Zimbabwe as compared to more developed countries.

2.6 Community, social and civic life

All participants considered it important to be reintegrated into the community. About 85% did not report any difficulty in participating in religious and spiritual activities and 95% considered them very important [32].

Fifty eight percent considered recreational activities as important. These recreational activities were mainly visiting friends and relatives, watching television, reading or listening to the radio [32]. There is a stark contrast in the type of recreational activities cited by the Zimbabwean sample as compared to other studies where participants reported restrictions in activities like golf, bowling, tennis and attending social clubs. The differences in the recreational activities can be explained by the differences in the socio-economic statuses of the samples. The culture of participating in recreational activities for leisure purposes need to be reinforced and further explored especially in low income groups where people mostly engage in productive activities whether paid or unpaid than they do in recreational activities.

2.7 Areas that stroke patients wanted to return to

Out of the 40 participants, 53% wanted to return to their work. They considered it very important because some were breadwinners and wanted to be able to look after their families [32]. In a study in Singapore by Kong and Yang [42], 14 out of 54 participants continued to be gainfully employed [42]. Of these 14, 11 were able to go back to previous jobs while 3 had to change jobs due to their physical limitations [42].

Thirty four percent wanted to be able to do their instrumental ADLs again [32]. These were mainly female participants who valued being able to look after their children and homes. Only 10% did not wish to return to any activity in particular and these were mainly elderly patients who had not been engaging in any activities that they considered important enough to return to [32]. In such cases, it would be necessary for the therapist to try to look for areas of interest for the patient so as to build a passion for doing activities that are meaningful to them and can also be used during therapy.

In summary, these findings give insight into the areas stroke patients consider important in the Zimbabwean context. They are consistent with other studies, for example, one study by Sumathipala [20], where stroke patients considered ADLs, social participation, mobility aids, home adaptations, housing and financial support as important [20].

The ICF is an important framework in guiding management of stroke patients as it can be used to assess and address all aspects of a person's life without just focusing on his/her diagnosis [43]. Occupational therapy has an important role of facilitating a patient's optimal functioning and independence through participation in meaningful and purposeful daily activities. The strength of occupational therapy lies in the ability to analyse activities/occupations. The occupations in which a person engages and the amount of time one spends doing the occupations is very specific to the circumstances and the culture in which a person lives [44]. Therefore, the effectiveness of occupational therapy and the quality of care can improve when culturally relevant occupations are selected and interventions are important to a person with stroke.

3. Needs of stroke patients

3.1 Introduction

This section is based on a cross sectional pilot study done in Harare, Zimbabwe in 2020 with 35 stroke patients attending rehabilitation [45]. Mean age of participants was 58 years (S.D 8.8) and the greater proportion were female (n = 19, 54.3%). The majority (94.3%) belonged to the Christian faith similar to 92% found in Seremwe *et al.* [46]'s study in the same context [46]. About 57% were married. In the Zimbabwean setting and from previous experiences with stroke patients, this might be due to good social and financial support from the spouse making them able to afford the hospital services. Those widowed or single due to other reasons may not seek for medical or rehabilitation services due to lack of financial and social support [46]. A study by Liu et al., [13] reported an independent association between marital status and post-stroke outcomes in patients with acute ischemic stroke [13].

About 49% were employed [45], consistent with another study done on stroke survivors in Zimbabwe where less than half were working and the rest had no source of income [46]. Left cerebral Vascular Accidents accounted for 74.3% of the strokes. Study participants had a median duration with stroke diagnosis of 104 days (inter-quartile range 44–270). This is mainly the situation in Zimbabwe where most of the patients who come for rehabilitation have stroke duration of less than two years. Those who had stroke for more than two years will have inadequate funds to continue treatment, hence will not come for rehabilitation services.

The needs of participants were grouped into physical, instrumental, social, informational and emotional needs. Highlighted in **Table 1** are the needs according to the groupings and it consists of 28 statements to which participants were expected to answer "yes" or "no" on whether they consider it a need.

3.2 Physical needs

Fourteen statements related to physical needs. All the participants in the study considered pain management, walking and general mobility, performing basic and instrumental activities of daily living (ADLs), engaging in recreational activities, dealing with fatigue and exercising as their physical needs post stroke [45]. Specific self-care needs cited were independent bathing and cutting toenails. Only 40% and about 11% cited swallowing and hearing problems respectively. Thus physical needs were the most common needs of stroke patients. This is because stroke mainly affects the physical components resulting in pain, reduced mobility, poor muscle strength, reduced speech and communication, problems with swallowing and incontinence and many other deficits which might results in decreased functioning and inability to cope [12]. In a similar study done in Australia, patients mostly over the age of 65 years needed assistance with performing ADLs, such as self-care [15], and this shows that this is a major need among all stroke patients regardless of location.

Sight problems, prevention of pressure sores and dealing with bladder and bowel problems were cited by more than 80% of participants as needs indicating that they are also common needs in this group.

3.3 Instrumental and social needs

These two aspects had a combined five needs (**Table 1**). There were two items on instrumental needs, and all participants indicated the need for additional

Item	Need	Considered as a need by stroke patients	
		Yes *n* (%)	No *n* (%)
	Physical needs		
1	To ease my pain, since nothing seems to ease it.	35 (100%)	0
2	Help on walking and general moving	35 (100%)	0
3	Help on how to get job done in my home (ADLs) such as cleaning, cooking, ironing and laundry	35 (100%)	0
4	Help on how to do things like cutting my toenails, washing myself	35 (100%)	0
5	Help on how to deal with fatigue	35 (100%)	0
6	Learning about exercise	35 (100%)	0
7	Help on how to bath independently	35 (100%)	0
8	Help on dealing with bladder/ bowel problems (accidents, constipation, diarrhoea)	32 (91.43%)	3 (8.57%)
9	Help on how to prevent pressure sores	30 (85.71)	5 (14.29%)
10	Help on sight problems.	29 (82.86%)	6 (17.14%)
11	Help on getting back to driving	19 (54.29%)	16 (45.71%)
12	Help on swallowing problems.	14 (40%)	21 (60%)
13	Help on speech and communication problems	12 (34.29%)	23 (65.71%)
14	Help on hearing problems.	4 (11.43%)	31 (88.57%)
	Instrumental support		
15	Additional aids or adaptations (kitchen appliances, stair lift, grab rails) if other please specify	35 (100%)	0
16	Adaptations outside the home (e.g., ramps, rail) if other please specify	33 (94.29%)	2 (5.71%)
	Social needs		
17	Help on how to occupy my day better (e.g., social outings, hobbies, leisure activities)	35 (100%)	0
18	Help and advocacy in accessing social services	34 (97.14%)	1 (2.86%)
19	Help on how to travel using public transport such as buses and commuter omnibuses	32 (91.43%)	3 (8.57%)
	Informational needs		
20	More information about my stroke (e.g., what is stroke, why has it happened to me, how to avoid having another one)	35 (100%)	0
21	Advice on how to improve my diet	35 (100%)	0
22	Advice on how to manage my money better.	33 (94.29%)	(5.71%)
23	Help on how to do shopping.	32 (91.43%)	3 (8.57%)
24	Advice on employment after stroke	25 (71.43%)	10 (28.57%)
25	Help and information on how to manage my physical relationship with my partner	13 (37.14%)	22 (62.86%)
	Emotional needs		
26	Help on improving self-esteem, anger issues and other emotional issues If other please specify	35 (100%)	0

Item	Need	Considered as a need by stroke patients	
		Yes *n* (%)	No *n* (%)
27	Help on improving my memory and concentration.	33 (94.29%)	2 (5.71%)
28	Help on how to deal with emotional and behavioural changes	34 (97.06%)	1 (2.94%)

Table 1.
Distribution of participants according to need (N = 35).

aids or adaptations in the house while 94% cited need for adaptations outside the home. Under social needs, there were three items and about 97 and 91% respectively indicated the need for help and advocacy in accessing social services and using public transport. All participants needed help on how to engage in social outings, hobbies and leisure activities. Stroke survivors in this study faced societal barriers that can affect engagement in activities of daily living namely problems in using public transportation, lack of adaptations inside and outside the home environment as well as lack of aids and appliances to facilitate independence. Due to the economic situation in Zimbabwe, most places are not specifically adapted for people with disabilities to engage fully in social and daily activities, for example, inadequate provision of rails and ramps in public buildings for those who have problems with mobility [47]. Assistive devices like wheelchairs and modifications to the home environment are not available to the survivor soon after discharge to promote maximum participation [48], hence participants citing them as needs they require occupational therapists to meet. In Zimbabwe, wheelchair service provision and services are fragmented and poorly integrated [49]. The use of mobility devices such as wheelchairs, crutches and canes improves mobility, health and quality of life, and it enables those with mobility issues to mobilise without any restrictions [48]. Another study showed that stroke survivors had more participation restrictions as a result of environmental barriers [50]. Physical/structural and services/assistance were considered the dominant barriers to participation in activities of daily life for stroke survivors in China, hence there were considered to be among the most common needs presented by stroke survivors [51]. In another study on "Identification of rehabilitation needs after a stroke", some of the most expressed needs of the participants were needs relating to adapted means of transportation and home visits from healthcare personnel [52]. Home visits might also help in noting any home adaptations that need to be done [53]. Social support should be provided to stroke survivors, including barrier-free facilities and occupational therapists should advocate for those services in the community.

3.4 Informational needs

Six items related to informational needs. All the participants needed information on their condition (stroke) and advice on diet. Over 90% needed advice on or help on better money management and shopping. Twenty-five participants needed advice on employment after stroke. The least cited as informational need had to do with managing physical relationships with partner/spouse (about 37%) (**Table 1**). The need to give more information about the condition is consistent with findings by Williams et al., where only 38% professed to know stroke warning signs and only 25% correctly interpreted their symptoms [54]. Similarly, Mckevitt, et al., reported more than half of their participants wanting more information about their stroke (cause, prevention of recurrence) [55]. This shows that this is a major concern among most stroke patients regardless of the part of the world they live, hence the need for occupational therapy intervention. Knowledge about the condition will also help them to adhere to the home programs they will be given and to seek for early treatment before any complications or permanent disability arises. With more knowledge about stroke, they could identify the disease immediately, resulting in a decrease in the time from symptom onset to hospital arrival, and a subsequent increase in the number of patients who may receive appropriate interventions [56]. It might also help them to know how to prevent any future recurrence of the condition and the services that might be beneficial to them in order to minimise any complications that may arise as a result of the condition.

3.5 Emotional needs

Three items related to emotional needs. All items were cited as needs by more than 94% (improving memory and concentration (94.29%), self-esteem, anger and other emotional issues (100%) plus dealing with the emotional and behavioural changes (97.06%) (**Table 1**). This high proportion of more than 90% of the participants having emotional needs after stroke is probably because stroke affects the person's ability to engage in daily living activities, communicate well with others and that can lead to increased dependence, feelings of low self-worth, (e.g., if the patient is incontinent) resulting in many psychological and emotional issues like depression [57]. The findings in this Zimbabwean study are consistent with a study on "Self-Reported Long-Term Needs After Stroke" where over one third of respondents reported experiencing emotional problems (including depression, crying) after the stroke [55]. Since emotional and psychological needs are liable to be neglected, post-stroke depression is a common complication which seriously impairs quality of life [18]. Therefore, psychological expertise and psychological support is needed by stoke survivors [18].

4. Importance of needs as perceived by stroke patients

The majority of the participants in the Zimbabwean study perceived most of the needs in all categories as important and requiring intervention [45]. Physical needs rated as very important in this study were independent mobility and dealing with bladder and bowel incontinence. These aspects enable participants to be independent and to perform daily activities without restrictions. Participants also perceived informational needs as important [45]. Information on dietary issues is important among stroke patients as this might enhance recovery and help in minimising the intake of unhealthy foods such as saturated fats and too much sodium chloride which might even increase the risk of having a recurrent stroke [58]. Knowledge about one's condition will conscientise them on the importance of receiving rehabilitation and adhering to one's treatment and medications. The knowledge can also minimise complications and prevent future recurrence of the condition, hence this information is important among stroke patients [59]. Furthermore, knowledge and information about the condition is important since there is often confusion and a lack of information about surviving after a stroke, prevention of subsequent strokes, treatment, services, benefits and adaptions to property [60, 61]. Stroke survivors had to adapt to changes in their bodies as a result of stroke and adjust their expectations, including roles within the home and community [60]. This was particularly so for those of working age and hence the importance of knowledge on the condition.

In one study, stroke survivors experienced a lack of information about what had happened to them and did not realise they had had a stroke [62]. Relevant information is required at different times after a stroke, for example, information about benefits and services most needed after discharge from hospital [61]. Some survivors and carers are unsure which profession offers which service, and there can be role confusion related to an Occupational Therapist, a Physiotherapist, a Home Carer and a social worker, hence this information is also important among stroke patients who should know which services can address their specific needs [60].

The majority of the patients in the Zimbabwean study indicated that adaptations in the home environment were important [45]. Without these, stroke survivors are restricted in performing their daily activities and social roles resulting in increased dependency [63]. Without assistive technology, stroke survivors and other people with disabilities are often excluded, isolated and locked into poverty, resulting in increased burden of morbidity and disability [63]. This is similar to a study done to identify the long-term needs of stroke survivors using the ICF where the participants reported that home adaptations (such as stair or grab rails) provided after discharge from hospital enabled them to adapt to their physical disabilities by facilitating independence in walking, climbing stairs and ADLs [20]. Stroke patients saw this as important since these factors might create a significant barrier to their physical functioning and independence.

Pfavai [45] also revealed that emotional issues such as dealing with depression and behavioural changes were rated as important by more than 80% of the participants. Most of these are not easily seen unlike physical needs hence their importance might be overlooked by occupational therapists. These issues might affect recovery and engagement in daily occupations hence they were perceived as important by the participants. Emotional problems such as depression might also be fatal, in worst cases leading to suicide and general increased mortality, hence their importance must not be overlooked [64]. A sudden attack and poor prognosis had an appreciable effect on the psychological and emotional wellbeing of stroke survivors [18], hence they are important and should be addressed. Interventions usually focus on treating the disease, rather than the emotional needs of the patients. These emotional and psychological needs are liable to be neglected and post-stroke depression is a common complication which seriously impairs quality of life [18, 63].

Participants in Zimbabwe also perceived the need to engage in recreational pursuits as important in their lives [45]. This is one of the areas which are mostly neglected during intervention by occupational therapists. However, engaging in leisure and recreational activities is of importance since it improves physical health, enhances mental wellness, social interaction with others and it enables the stroke survivors to engage in activities which are meaningful in their lives [65]. In a study done on coping with the challenges of recovering from stroke, participants reported the importance of recreational activities and the great distress which was associated with the loss of hobbies and activities that had previously been a source of pleasure and achievement [62]. This is also in line with Rhoda et al., [66] where the participants highlighted the importance of engaging in recreational activities. Participants experienced social isolation, restriction to their homes which they felt could result in sadness and depression due to inability to engage in those activities which were normally found interesting before [66]. However, these activities should be client centred so that their benefits to each individual can be realised.

Access to public transport which is conducive and specifically adapted for people with disabilities was perceived as important by participants in Pfavai study [45]. This is important since lack of suitable transport results in participation restriction in activities such as religious activities, shopping and other social gatherings participants might want to engage in [47]. In a study done in China, physical/structural and services/assistance which include inaccessible public transport for those with disabilities were considered the dominant barriers to participation in activities of daily life for stroke survivors in China hence these needs are important and should be addressed [18]. Social support should be provided to stroke survivors, including barrier-free facilities [47]. Furthermore, the social security system for stroke survivors and other disabling conditions needs to be improved in low-income and middle-income countries.

5. Perceived fulfilment of stroke patients' needs

Findings from Pfavai study [45] indicated that most of the needs of stroke patients were not being fully met including those needs participants rated as very important. Perceived unmet needs may reflect expectations and knowledge but may also indicate where service provision should be developed [55]. The needs which were mostly being fulfilled were physical needs such as pain management, exercises to facilitate walking and mobility in general, and self-care including independent bathing [45]. This is because these needs can be easily identified and their physical limitations can be easily noted compared to other needs such as emotional, informational and societal. The later ones are therefore less likely to be addressed. These findings are consistent with McKevitt *et al.*, [55] where most participants experienced problems related to physical needs which were to do with mobility, falls, pain, and incontinence, and those needs were fulfilled in the majority of cases. Thus, the percentages of those with unmet physical needs were small (less than 25%) compared to the unmet emotional needs such as memory and concentration which were reported by 39% of the participants [55].

The emotional needs highlighted included how to deal with depression, anger issues, low self-esteem and behavioural changes as a result of stroke [45]. Emotional needs might be overlooked during the assessment process especially if the patient does not mention any emotional issues they might be experiencing. This is in line with a study done on the unmet needs of stroke patients where cognitive and emotional health needs such as concentration, memory, cognition, fatigue, and emotions were less likely to be fully met than physical needs despite physical needs being more common [15]. This affirms the requirement to implement strategies to help stroke survivors address the range of emotional problems they may experience [55]. Stroke rehabilitation usually focuses on physical impairments and assisting stroke survivors to develop functional independence. This may mean that services aimed at addressing the cognitive and emotional needs of stroke survivors are not adequately resourced [15]. This supports the results obtained in Pfavai [45] study where emotional needs were not being fully met compared to most of the physical needs [45]. Therapists need to be intentional in ensuring that emotional problems experienced by stroke survivors are adequately addressed.

Instrumental needs which were perceived as being unmet by more than 70% of the participants included adaptations outside the home environment and aids and adaptions inside the home environment [45]. Without these aids, stroke survivors are less able to perform their daily activities without restrictions [49]. However, due to the economic situation in Zimbabwe there is lack of resources in hospitals and assistive devices are scarce for those with performance limitations [45, 47]. There is also lack of transport and financial resources for the occupational therapists to do home adaptations for the patients soon after discharge [53]. This need might also be more than the 70% which was obtained in Pfavai study [45] since the study was partly done at a rehabilitation centre where the patients are given assistive devices such as wheelchairs for them to use before discharge and at a nominal fee after discharge. Stroke survivors have also reported that health systems are not responsive to their changing needs and that there is a lack of long-term re-assessment of their needs, [15]; hence some of the needs which might arise later during intervention may not be met.

Training on getting back to driving and information on how to do shopping were rated by more than 90% of participants as unmet [45]. These are some of the needs which are over looked during intervention. This might be due to lack of expertise among the concerned occupational therapists on driving rehabilitation. At the time of writing this chapter, there was no comprehensive module on driving in the University of Zimbabwe curriculum on occupational therapy undergraduate training. This might result in lack of expertise and confidence in addressing that need. This is also in line with a study done on coping with the challenges of recovering from stroke where loss of ability to drive a car was seen as a major challenge which required intervention and the ability to resume driving was spoken with deep emotion [62]. Driving was seen as representative of independence, a way to regain self-esteem, a means to access social support and to facilitate participation in valued activities [62]. This aspect however needs special training to avoid causing harm to patient and society.

Skills on shopping independently were also perceived as unmet in Pfavai study [45], and this might be due to lack of resources to simulate the shopping environment or lack of funds to teach the patients in the actual environment. In a study that looked at the combined perceptions of people with stroke and their carers regarding rehabilitation needs one year after stroke [67], patients reported having to give up a task in advance and had limitations in more physically demanding activities such as going to buy groceries among other tasks, supporting the need to address shopping needs among stroke patients [67]. The importance of this need might be overlooked during interventions. Information and knowledge needs of stroke survivors should not be underestimated and should be considered when developing strategies to meet the rehabilitation needs of stroke survivors [68].

Another unmet need in the Zimbabwean study [45] was financial/money management after a stroke. Most stroke survivors lose their jobs after the incident of stroke, and cognitive components might also be affected resulting in inability to adequately manage their money. However, this need seemed to have been overlooked. Li et al. also noted that few studies have looked at the financial impact of stroke on the survivors and their families, indicating that this area's importance might be underrated [18].

Early discharge of patients due to unavailability of beds might also result in some of the stroke patients' needs not being adequately met. Although many individuals still have rehabilitation needs one year after stroke, rehabilitation is often concluded within the first three months, and follow up is not usually done hence some of the needs might not be adequately fulfilled [67].

6. Closing remarks

The occupational therapist is the health professional who specifically addresses patients' involvement in daily life situations, and as such, she/he should be well conversant with that particular aspect of patients' lives. This in turn addresses one's quality of life which is often neglected. Stroke patients' perceived needs highlighted above provide patients' perspectives which is critical in the development of patient-centred services by service providers. The commonly used functional outcome measures (e.g., the Barthel Index) may underestimate dependence leading to rehabilitation professionals and patients prioritising different needs. Not using meaningful occupations in treatment; lack of discharge planning, using interventions not perceived as driven by patient's occupational goals, and use of interventions chosen by therapists without considering what the patient needs thereby placing the patient in a passive role were noted as major challenges [69]. The stroke patients' perceptions help the therapists to tailor interventions to meet patients' specific needs.

Author details

Tecla Mlambo[1*], Yvonne Pfavai[1], Faith R. Chimusoro[2] and Farayi Kaseke[1]

1 University of Zimbabwe, Harare, Zimbabwe

2 Ministry of Health and Child Care, Zimbabwe

*Address all correspondence to: teclamlambo@hotmail.com

IntechOpen

References

[1] Gund BM. Stroke: A brain attack. IOSR Journal of Pharmacy. 2013;**03**(08):1-23

[2] Sacco RL, Kasner SE, Broderick JP, Caplan LR, Connors JJ, Culebras A, et al. An updated definition of stroke for the 21st century: A statement for healthcare professionals from the American Heart Association/American Stroke Association. Stroke. 2013;**44**(7):2064-2089

[3] Johnson W, Onuma O, Owolabi M, Sachdev S. Stroke: A global response is needed. Bulletin of the World Health Organization. 2016;**94**(9):634A-635A

[4] Kalavina R. The challenges and experiences of stroke patients and their spouses in Blantyre, Malawi. Malawi Medical Journal. 2019;**31**(2):112

[5] Wittenauer R, Smith L. Background paper 6.6 ischaemic and haemorrhagic stroke. In: Priority Medicines For Europe and "The World" A Public Health Approach To Innovation. 2012 https://docplayer.net/23829358-Background-paper-6-6-ischaemic-and-haemorrhagic-stroke.html. [Accessed: 15 November 2021]

[6] Johnson CO, Nguyen M, Roth GA, Nichols E, Alam T, Abate D, et al. Global, regional, and national burden of stroke, 1990-2016: A systematic analysis for the Global Burden of Disease Study 2016. The Lancet Neurology. 2019;**18**(5):439-458

[7] Kaseke F, Stewart A, Gwanzura L, Hakim J, Chikwasha V. Clinical characteristics and outcomes of patients with stroke admitted to three tertiary hospitals in Zimbabwe: A retrospective one-year study. Malawi Medical Journal. 2017;**29**(June):177-182

[8] Darkhabani Z. Stroke and TIA Assessment and Management. Dallas, Texas: American Heart Association;

2008 Available from: https://www.heart.org/idc/groups/heart-public/@wcm/@mwa/documents/downloadable/ucm_467064.pdf

[9] Ekeh BC. Challenges of the management of stroke in Sub Saharan Africa: Evaluating awareness, access and action. Journal of Pediatric Neurology. 2017;**02**(03):1-6

[10] Stroke Association Emotional changes after stroke. 2012:1-12. https://www.google.co.zw/url?sa=t&rct=j&q=&esrc=s&source=web&cd=&ved=2ahUKEwi_o-K11p30AhUI3KQKHVF-CuAQFnoECAkQAQ&url=http%3A%2F%2Fwww.stroke.org.uk%2Fsites%2Fdefault%2Ffiles%2FEmotional%2520changes%2520after%2520stroke.pdf&usg=AOvVaw2wkfBKuAwgYZY56NrPpBVd

[11] Welters K. Current Trends in Occupational Therapy Treatment for People with Stroke. Tacoma, Washington: University of Puget Sound; 2011

[12] Cawood J, Visagie S. Stroke management and functional outcomes of stroke survivors in an urban Western Cape Province setting. South African Journal of Occupational Therapy. 2016;**46**(3):21-26

[13] Lui S, Nguyen MH. Elderly stroke rehabilitation: Overcoming the complications. HIndawi. 2018;**2018**:1-9

[14] Goldstein LB, Bushnell CD, Adams RJ, Appel LJ, Braun LT, Chaturvedi S, et al. Guidelines for the primary prevention of stroke: A guideline for healthcare professionals from the American Heart Association/American Stroke Association. Stroke. 2011;**42**(2):517-584

[15] Andrew NE, Kilkenny M, Naylor R, Purvis T, Lalor E, Moloczij N, et al.

Understanding long-term unmet needs in Australian survivors of stroke. International Journal of Stroke. 2014;9(A100):106-112

[16] Ullberg T, Zia E, Petersson J, Norrving B. Perceived unmet rhabilitation needs 1 year after stroke: An observational study from the Swedish stroke register. Stroke. 2016;47(2):539-541. DOI: 10.1161/STROKEAHA.115.011670

[17] Hsieh M-C, Hwang C-L, Jeng J-S, Wang J-S. Estimation of the long-term care needs of stroke patients by integrating functional disability and survival. PLoS One. 2013;8(10):75605 Available from: www.plosone.org

[18] Li X, Xia X, Wang P, et al. Needs and rights awareness of stroke survivors and caregivers: A cross-sectional, single-centre questionnaire survey. BMJ Open. 2017;7(10):e013210. DOI: 10.1136/bmjopen-2016-013210

[19] Reed M, Harrington R, Duggan Á, Wood VA. Meeting stroke survivors perceived needs: A qualitative study of a community-based exercise and education scheme. Clinical Rehabilitation. 2010;24(1):16-25

[20] Sumathipala K, Radcliffe E, Sadler E, Wolfe CDA, McKevitt C. Identifying the long-term needs of stroke survivors using the International classification of functioning, disability and health. Chronic Illness. 2012;8(1):31-44

[21] Hebert D, Lindsay MP, McIntyre A, Kirton A, Rumney PG, Bagg S, et al. Canadian stroke best practice recommendations: Stroke rehabilitation practice guidelines, update 2015. International Journal of Stroke. 2016;11(4):459-484

[22] Laughton F, O'Toole J, Robertson L. Stroke: Emergency Care and Rehabilitation. https://www.google. co.zw/url?sa=t&rct=j&q=&esrc=s&source=web&cd=&ved=2ahUKEwiEzPvknp30AhVMCewKHbF1DjUQFnoECAcQAQ&url=https%3A%2F%2Fwww.atrainceu.com%2Fsites%2Fdefault%2Ffiles%2FStroke-Print%2520and%2520Go.pdf&usg=AOvVaw2WVybGmTXl16GAiHSOcshw. [Accessed: 16 November 2021]

[23] Rowland T, Cooke D, Gustafsson L. Role of occupational therapy after stroke. Annals of Indian Academy of Neurology. 2008;11(Suppl. 5):99-107

[24] Pulaski KH. Adult neurological dysfunction. In: Crepeau EB, Cohn ES, BAB S, editors. Willard and Spackman's Occupational Therapy. Philadelphia: Lippincott and Williams and Wilkins; 2003

[25] Kielhofner. Model of Human Occupation. Philadelphia: Lippincott Williams and Wilkins; 2008

[26] WHO. International classification of functioning, health and disability. 2001 World Health Organization, Geneva, Switzerland

[27] Abarghuei AF, Mehraban AH, Yousefi M. The clinical application of ICF model for occupational therapy in a patient with stroke: A case report. Medical Journal of the Islamic Republic of Iran. 2018;32(65):381-385

[28] Mpofu E, Oakland T. Rehabilitation and Health Assessment. 3rd ed. New York: Springer Publishing Company; 2009

[29] WFOT. Statement on occupational therapy. World Federation of Occupational Therapists. 2010;1(1):1. Available from: http://www.wfot.org/Portals/0/PDF/STATEMENT ON OCCUPATIONAL THERAPY 300811.pdf%5Cn; http://bjo.sagepub.com/lookup/doi/10.4276/030802214X14018723137959%5Cn; http://www.england.nhs.uk/wp-content/uploads/2013/06/

c03-med-low-sec-mh.pdf%5Cn;
http://hdl.handle.net/24

[30] Olsson L, Lundborg M.
Occupational Therapy Process for
Patients after Stroke in Thailand.
Örebro, Sweden: Örebro
University; 2015

[31] Tistad M, Tham K, von Koch L,
Ytterberg C. Unfulfilled rehabilitation
needs and dissatisfaction with care 12
months after a stroke: An explorative
observational study. BMC Neurology.
2012;**18**:12

[32] Chimusoro FR. Activities and
Participation Domains Considered
Important by Stroke Patients Attending
Rehabilitation in Harare. Zimbabwe
[Harare]: University of Zimbabwe; 2012

[33] Chimusoro FR, Mlambo T. Activities
and participation domains considered
important by stroke patients attending
rehabilitation in Harare, Zimbabwe.
Central African Journal of Medicine.
2013;**59**(9/12):20

[34] Mlambo T, Amosun SL, Concha M.
Timing of occupational therapy services
in the rehabilitation of stroke patients in
an academic hospital in South Africa.
South African Journal of Occupational
Therapy. 2006;**36**(2):5-8

[35] Trombly Latham CA, Radomski MV.
Occupational Therapy for Physical
Dysfunction. 5th ed. Philadelphia:
Lippincott Williams and Wilkins; 2008

[36] Pedretti LW, Early MB.
Occupational Practice Skills for Physical
Dysfunction. 5th ed. Missouri:
Mosby; 2001

[37] Kneebone II, Lincoln NB.
Psychological problems after stroke and
their management: State of knowledge.
Neuroscience and Medicine.
2012;**03**(01):83-89

[38] Duncan PW, Zorowitz R, Bates B,
Choi JY, Glasberg JJ, Graham GD.
Management of adult stroke
rehabilitation care. A clinical practice
guideline*.AHA/ASA-Endorsed practice
guidelines. Stroke. 2005;**36**(9):
e100-e143. DOI: 10.1161/01.
STR.0000180861.54180.FF

[39] Åberg AC, Sidenvall B,
Hepworth M, O'Reilly K, Lithell H. On
loss of activity and independence,
adaptation improves life satisfaction in
old age–a qualitative study of patients'
perceptions. Quality of Life Research.
2005;**14**(4):1111-1125

[40] Edmans J. Occupational Therapy
and Stroke. United Kingdom:
Wiley-Blackwell; 2011

[41] D'Alisa S, Baudo S, Mauro A,
Miscio G. How does stroke restrict
participation in the long term post
stroke survivors. Acta Neurologica
Scandinavica. 2005;**12**(3):157-162

[42] Kong KH, Yang SY. Health-related
quality of life among chronic stroke
survivors attending a rehabilitation
clinic. Singapore Medical Journal.
2006;**47**(3):213-218

[43] WHO. Towards a Common
Language for Functioning, Disability
and Health ICF Towards a Common
Language for Functioning, Disability
and Health: ICF The International
Classification of Functioning, Disability
and Health. Geneva: World Health
Organization; 2002

[44] Crouch R. The relationship between
culture and occupation in Africa. In:
Occupational Therapy: An African
Perspective. Johannesburg: Camera
Press; 2010

[45] Pfavai Y. Needs of Stroke Patients
and Their Perceived Fulfilment of these
Needs in Occupational Therapy. Harare,
Zimbabwe: University of
Zimbabwe; 2020

[46] Seremwe F, Kaseke F,
Chikwanha TM, Chikwasha V. Factors

associated with hospital arrival time after the onset of stroke symptoms: A cross-sectional study at two teaching hospitals in Harare, Zimbabwe. Malawi Medical Journal. 2017;**29**(2):171. DOI: 10.4314/mmj.v29i2.18

[47] Munemo E. Accessibility of public and private amenities for people with disabilities in the Central Business District of Harare. Advances in Social Sciences Research Journal. 2018;**5**(10): 276-288

[48] Rohwerder B. Assistive technologies in developing countries. In: K4D Helpdesk Report. Brighton, UK: Institute of Development Studies; 2018

[49] Visagie S, Mlambo T, Van der Veen J, Nhunzvi C, Tigere D, Scheffler E. Is any wheelchair better than no wheelchair? A Zimbabwean perspective. African Journal of Disability. 2015;**4**(1):1-10

[50] Skolarus LE, Burke FJ, Brown DL, Freedman VA. Understanding stroke survivorship: Expanding the concept of poststroke disability. Stroke. 2014;**45**(1):224-230

[51] Zhang L, Yan T, You L, Li K. Barriers to activity and participation for stroke survivors in rural China. Archives of Physical Medicine and Rehabilitation. 2015;**96**(7):1222-1228

[52] Talbot LR, Viscogliosi C, Desrosiers J, Vincent C, Rousseau J, Robichaud L. Identification of rehabilitation needs after a stroke: An exploratory study. Health and Quality of Life Outcomes. 2004;**21**:2

[53] Dangarembizi N, Mlambo T, Chinengo TPT. Home visits by occupational therapists in Zimbabwe: The extent and challenges. Central African Journal of Medicine. 2011;**57**:S18

[54] Williams LS, Bruno A, Rouch D, Marriott DJ, MAS. Stroke patients'

knowledge of stroke: Influence on time to presentation. Stroke. 1997;**28**(5):912-915

[55] McKevitt C, Fudge N, Redfern J, Sheldenkar A, Crichton S, Rudd AR, et al. Self-reported long-term needs after stroke. Stroke. 2011;**42**(5):1398-1403

[56] Hachinski V, Donnan GA, Gorelick PB, Hacke W, Cramer SC, Kaste M, et al. Stroke: Working toward a prioritized world agenda. Stroke. 2010;**41**(6):1084-1099

[57] Kniepmann K. Female family carers for survivors of stroke: Occupational loss and quality of life. British Journal of Occupational Therapy. 2012;**75**(5): 208-216

[58] Foroughi M, Akhavanzanjani M, Maghsoudi Z, Ghiasvand R, Khorvash F, Askari G. Stroke and nutrition: A review of studies. International Journal of Preventive Medicine. Isfahan University of Medical Sciences (IUMS). 2013;**4**:S165-S179 Available from: /pmc/ articles/PMC3678213/?report=abstract

[59] Soto-Cámara R, González-Bernal JJ, González-Santos J, Aguilar-Parra JM, Trigueros R, López-Liria R. Knowledge on signs and risk factors in stroke patients. Journal of Clinical Medicine. 2020;**9**(8):2557. DOI: 10.3390/ jcm9082557

[60] Hare R, Rogers H, Lester H, McManus R, Mant J. What do stroke patients and their carers want from community services? Family Practice. 2006;**23**(1):131-136

[61] Mackenzie A, Perry L, Lockhart E, Cottee M, Cloud G, Mann H. Family carers of stroke survivors: Needs, knowledge, satisfaction and competence in caring. Disability and Rehabilitation. 2007;**29**(2):111-121

[62] Ch'ng AM, French D, McLean N. Coping with the challenges of recovery

from stroke: Long term perspectives of stroke support group members. Journal of Health Psychology. 2008;**13**(8): 1136-1146

[63] World Health Organization. Seventy-First World Health Assembly Improving Access to Assistive Rechnology The Need For Assistive Technology 2. Geneva, Switzerland: World Health Organization; 2018 Available from: http://www.who.int/ disabilities/publications/technology/ wheelchairguidelines/en

[64] Dar K, Venigalla H, Khan AM, Ahmed R, Mekala HM, Zain H, et al. Post stroke depression frequently overlooked, undiagnosed, untreated. Neuropsychiatry (London). 2017;**07**(06):906-919

[65] Yi TI, Han JS, Lee KE, Ha SA. Participation in leisure activity and exercise of chronic stroke survivors using community-based rehabilitation services in Seongnam City. Annals of Rehabilitation Medicine. 2015;**39**(2):234-242

[66] Rhoda A, Cunningham N, Azaria S, Urimubenshi G. Provision of inpatient rehabilitation and challenges experienced with participation post discharge: Quantitative and qualitative inquiry of African stroke patients. BMC Health Services Research. 2015;**15**(1): 1-9. DOI: 10.1186/s12913-015-1057-z

[67] Ekstam L, Johansson U, Guidetti S, Eriksson G, Ytterberg C. The combined perceptions of people with stroke and their carers regarding rehabilitation needs 1 year after stroke: A mixed methods study. BMJ Open. 2015;5(2):1-8

[68] Kamalakannan S, Gudlavalleti Venkata M, Prost A, Natarajan S, Pant H, Chitalurri N, et al. Rehabilitation needs of stroke survivors after discharge from hospital in India. Archives of Physical Medicine and Rehabilitation. 2016;**97**:1526-1532.e9

Available from: http://creativecommons. org/licenses/by/4.0/

[69] Boutin-Lester P, Gibson RW. Patients' perceptions of home health occupational therapy. Australian Occupational Therapy Journal. 2002;**49**(3):146-154